THE DEVELOPING HEART: A 'HISTORY' OF PEDIATRIC CARDIOLOGY

Developments in Cardiovascular Medicine

VOLUME 163

The Developing Heart: A 'History' of Pediatric Cardiology

by

CATHERINE A. NEILL
Professor Emeritus,
Johns Hopkins Medical Institutions,
Baltimore, MD, U.S.A.

and

EDWARD B. CLARK
Professor of Pediatrics,
Rochester School of Medicine,
Rochester, NY, U.S.A.

KLUWER ACADEMIC PUBLISHERS
DORDRECHT / BOSTON / LONDON

Library of Congress Cataloging-in-Publication Data

The developing heart : a 'history' of pediatric cardiology / edited by
Catherine A. Neill and Edward B. Clark.
p. cm. -- (Developments in cardiovascular medicine ; v. 163)
Includes bibliographical references and index.
ISBN 0-7923-3375-6(HB : alk. paper)
1. Pediatric cardiology--History. I. Neill, Catherine A.
II. Clark, Edward B. III. Series.
[DNLM: 1. Heart Diseases--in infancy & childhood. 2. Heart
Surgery--in infancy & childhood. 3. Cardiology--trends. W1
DE997VME v.163 1995 / WS 290 D489 1995]
RJ421.D48 1995
618.92'12'009--dc20
DNLM/DLC
for Library of Congress 95-3082

ISBN 0-7923-3375-6

Published by Kluwer Academic Publishers,
P.O. Box 17, 3300 AA Dordrecht, The Netherlands.

Kluwer Academic Publishers incorporates
the publishing programmes of
D. Reidel, Martinus Nijhoff, Dr W. Junk and MTP Press.

Sold and distributed in the U.S.A. and Canada
by Kluwer Academic Publishers,
101 Philip Drive, Norwell, MA 02061, U.S.A.

In all other countries, sold and distributed
by Kluwer Academic Publishers Group,
P.O. Box 322, 3300 AH Dordrecht, The Netherlands.

Illustrations by Timothy H. Phelps M.S., CMI, FAMI

Typesetting by Frances Weber, The Type House, Baltimore

Cover:
design Timothy H. Phelps
photography Jim Durham, medical photographer
type design Joseph M. Dieter, Jr.

Printed on acid-free paper

Printed in the Netherlands

CONTENTS

FOREWORD

THE DEVELOPING HEART: A "HISTORY" OF PEDIATRIC CARDIOLOGY

"Le Coeur a ses raisons ..."

"L'homme n'est qu'un roseau ... mais c'est un roseau pensant.
(Man is a reed ... but a thinking reed).
—Pensees de Blaise Pascal

Pediatric cardiology is the study of the heart of a child. The decade of the 1990s marks the 50th anniversary of the beginning of surgery for children's hearts. The aura of celebration surrounding this anniversary, the end of a vivid and heroic age, together with the rapid approach of the 21st century, makes this a propitious time to consider the history of pediatric cardiology.

A historian of pediatric cardiology could tackle a number of fascinating questions. When was childhood heart disease first recognised? What civilisation first studied the fetal heart? Have all the cardiac pioneers been given their just appreciation? And, although children have always had hearts, why is pediatric cardiology so new? Indeed, is it so new that a "history" is premature?

In this brief overview we will address these questions obliquely, focusing on the growth of knowledge of pediatric cardiology, particularly in the last half century. The growth of knowledge has varied in different decades, but has always been incremental, building on past discoveries. This is a vital and evolving field. Knowledge has moved from anatomic concepts, through physiology, diagnosis and effective therapy, to the present era when cardiac development comes of age.

A number of excellent vignettes and biographies of some of the great cardiologists and surgeons are available. Our study will consider the 4 eras of pediatric cardiology, the gradual growth of knowledge prior to this century, the explosive developments of the last 50 years, and some of the problems beginning to be recognised in the new and current "developmental era." Growth in knowledge has been both episodic and dramatic, yet it would be wrong to present a picture of unalloyed achievement.

A major theme in the four eras concerns the interaction of tools and concepts in the growth of knowledge. Sometimes a major concept preceded a tool of study; a striking example is Fick's concept of cardiac output, preceding by many years the tool of the cardiac catheter needed for measurement and validation of the concept. Another theme is the role of the pioneers, and particularly which tools and concepts were involved in their pioneering efforts. Two women, Maude Abbott and Helen Taussig, were major pioneers, and other women have worked and contributed actively to pediatric cardiology since it was first defined.

Another important topic, one which will be added to greatly by future historians, concerns the little we know of the child with heart disease through the ages. Before saying more of history, the field of pediatric cardiology needs to be defined.

INTRODUCTION

The twentieth century has seen extraordinary changes in the understanding and treatment of cardiac malformations, changes so profound that pediatric cardiology is sometimes thought of as concerned only with the diagnosis and management of congenital heart defects. Although the discipline was identified, named, and grew during the time these dramatic changes were occurring, pediatric cardiology is not confined to the malformed heart. It also involves the healthy heart before and after birth, and the preservation of heart health into adult life. Table 1 summarises the four domains of pediatric cardiology.

Table 1
THE 4 DOMAINS OF PEDIATRIC CARDIOLOGY

- **The Developing Heart**
- **Normal Heart and Circulation**
- **Heart Defects and Childhood Heart Disease**
- **Preventive Cardiology**

Each of these four domains has its own history, since the timing of advances and the rate of growth of knowledge in each domain has differed. The study of the normal heart has a much longer and more complex history than that of childhood heart disease, yet the histories of all four domains have interacted and influenced each other. For example, many of the techniques now used to study the developing heart use methods first elaborated in the normal heart of men and larger animals.

The Developing Heart

Many different disciplines are now involved in the study of the embryonic growth of the heart, ranging from molecular biology through fetal Doppler-echocardiography, teratology and hemodynamics. Some of these approaches are very new, beginning only in this century. Although the beating of the embryonic chick heart has been described at least since the time of Aristotle, modern cardiac embryology had to await the discovery of such tools as the microscope, and the concepts of fetal physiology.

The Normal Heart and Circulation

The four chambers of the normal heart have been recognised since ancient times, but our current understanding of the normal heart and circulation has taken many centuries. The modern concept of the 2 circulations dates from William Harvey. The publication of his monograph De Motu Cordis in 1628 [1] is used by most cardiac historians as a dividing point separating the era of ancient concepts of the circulation from those current today.

Heart Defects and Childhood Heart Disease

Anatomic cardiac defects began to be described in the 17th century, with the growth of the disciplines of anatomy and pathology. However, the detailed study of children's hearts began in the 20th century. At the beginning of this century, understanding was primarily an exercise in anatomy and pathology. Acquired heart problems were a greater focus of clinical study in children than congenital defects. When Helen Taussig became Director of the Children's Heart Clinic at Johns Hopkins Hospital Baltimore in 1932, rheumatic heart disease was still a major scourge. Helen Taussig's mentor, Dr Edwards A Park, urged her to study congenital cardiac malformations, then considered a rare and discouraging problem. Following the advent of cardiac surgery and cardiac catheterisation in the 1940s explosive changes occurred in diagnosis and management of heart defects. Systematic study of childhood arrhythmias and cardiomyopathies, and the recognition of Kawasaki disease, followed many decades after pediatric cardiology had become accepted as a growing and vital discipline.

Preventive Cardiology

The 4th domain of pediatric cardiology concerns efforts to maintain the healthy heart of a child into adult life and old age. It is axiomatic, if seldom acknowledged, that every adult once had the heart of a child, indeed once had an embryonic and then a fetal heart. A number of "adult" heart problems may well have their beginnings in very early life. Even from ancient times, exercise, moderation in eating, and a healthy life style have been urged by physiscians and philosophers as a recipe for a long and happy life. The term "preventive cardiology" however, only began to be used in the literature on coronary atherosclerosis in the early 1950s, and became part of conceptual thinking in pediatric cardiology somewhat later, in the early 1960s.

Just as the modern era of heart surgery began with the treatment of pediatric heart disease, so are researchers in coronary heart disease and hypertension increasingly concerned with a search for precursors. In this history we will stress the ultimate unity of approaches to knowledge of children's hearts.

THE FOUR ERAS OF PEDIATRIC CARDIOLOGY

At the beginning of this century many forms of congenital and acquired heart disease had been described, and some physiologic consequences were known. Clinico-physiologic profiles for certain defects, such as patent ductus arteriosus, were widely recognised by the 1940s. Nevertheless, until surgery became available, heart disease in children was thought of mainly as an academic challenge, of intellectual and pathologic interest only. The publication of Maude Abbott's Atlas of Congenital Cardiac Disease in 1936[2] was closely followed in time by the advent of heart surgery and cardiac catheterisation. We have used the date of publication of her Atlas to mark the culmination of the first era of pediatric cardiology, **the era of pathologic anatomy** (Figure 1).

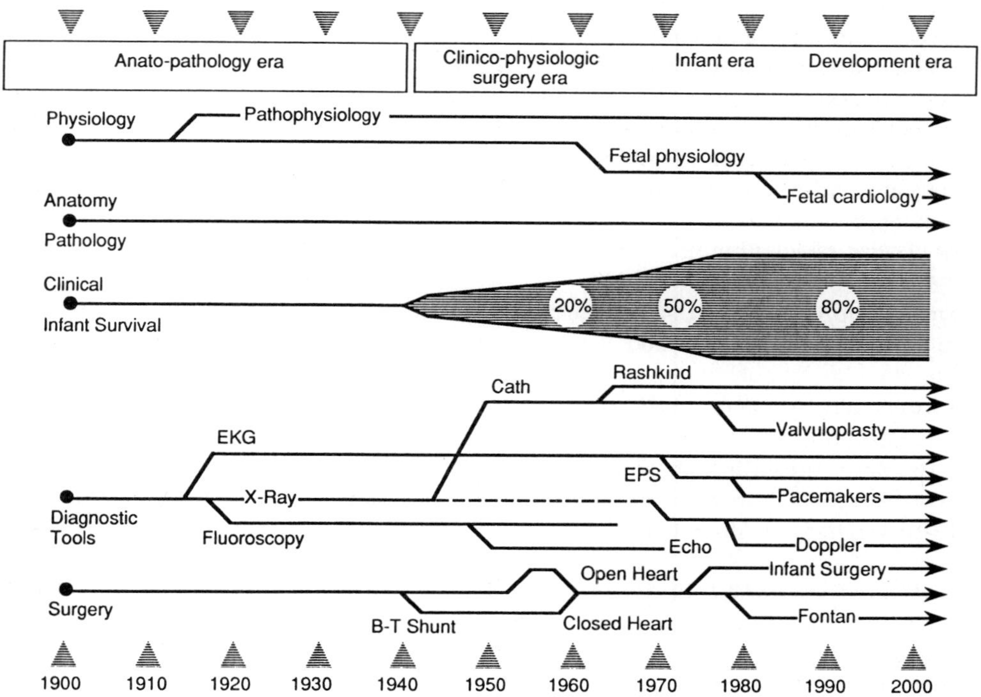

Figure 1—The 4 eras of pediatric cardiology, showing the timing of introduction of some new tools and concepts. The survival of infants born with heart defects has improved markedly during the past half century.

The Era of Clinicophysiologic Correlations and Surgery, beginning in the late 1930s and early 1940s marked the onset of the new therapeutic age, characterised by many rapid advances. The era began with closed heart surgery, ligation of a patent ductus, the Blalock Taussig shunt procedure, and coarctation repair, all described between 1939 and 1945. The advent of therapy heralded a remarkable upsurge in diagnostic techniques, accompanied by a rapid widening of operative approaches. Collaborative teams of pediatricians, physiologists, radiologists and surgeons grew worldwide.

Successful open heart surgery began in the mid 1950s, and by the mid 1970s the discipline of pediatric cardiology was well established. Studies of natural history and of heart disease in infancy, including the New England Regional Infant Cardiac study, were accompanied by technical surgical advances, so that by the mid 1970s a new era dawned.

The Infant Era began in the mid 1970s, with the spread of early diagnosis and successful surgical therapy in infancy. Changes were greatly accelerated by the arrival of new technologies, including echocardiography, improvements in myocardial preservation and surgical techniques, and the advent of prostaglandin therapy. As echocardiography became increasingly sophisticated, accurate neonatal and even prenatal diagnosis became possible at the bedside. Doppler echocardiography, for the first time in history, allowed simultaneous visualisation of both intracardiac anatomy and physiology. Many advances, including fetal echocardiography, allowed new approaches to the developing heart, and ushered in the present era of studies of cardiac development.

The Developmental Era, starting around 1990, has already seen remarkable advances in understanding normal and abnormal cardiac development. To use but one example, the clinical correlation of Down syndrome with atrioventricular canal had been appreciated by Maude Abbott in the early decades of this century, and Lejeune's recognition in the 1950s of trisomy 21 as the genetic basis of Down syndrome was a dramatic breakthrough. Only now, by use of the sophisticated tools of genetic analysis available in the 1990s, is the molecular basis of the association beginning to be understood. Molecular biologic approaches to heart problems are very recent.

The Four Eras and Tetralogy of Fallot. This defect occupies a prominent and intriguing role in the history of pediatric cardiology. In the era of pathologic anatomy, many detailed reports were made of the anatomic findings, and some early clinicophysiologic correlations had begun. The clinical profile of "typical" tetralogy was known in outline by the late 1930s, but was of little interest to most cardiologists and pediatricians, since such knowledge had no attendant therapy. The term "blue baby," echoing the phrase "blue boy" used by Sandifort to describe his patient in the eighteenth century, was still sometimes used by physicians. It sounded dark and mysterious, a term adequate enough to convey a confusing and untreatable disorder.

The advent of the Blalock Taussig shunt in 1944, ushering in the clinicophysiologic era, revolutionised thinking about tetralogy, and indeed all forms of heart disease. As children were turned from "blue to pink," a phrase often used by Helen Taussig, the dark shadow of incurability was lifted from the "morbus caeruleus" [3] which included tetralogy of Fallot as its most frequent anomaly. Subsequent follow up studies, and the growth of cardiac catheterisation and angiocardiography, led to understanding of hemodynamics and the effects of hypoxemia.

After open heart repair began in the 1950s, increasing numbers of patients reached adulthood, and interest shifted to their subsequent quality of life, and to long term surgical sequelae. In the infant era, from the mid 1970s onwards, early noninvasive diagnosis was increasingly often followed by primary intracardiac repair in the first year of life.

Now, in the developmental era, the focus of research is turning to the question so long of interest to patients, parents and families, the question of etiology. Recent molecular biologic studies of the CATCH22 syndrome give hope for early understanding of the genetic mechanisms behind this cardiac disorder which has been so famous in the history of pediatric cardiology in all 4 eras. (Table 2)

Table 2
The 4 Eras of Pediatric Cardiology

• **Pathologic anatomy era culminating in Abbott Atlas**	**1936**
• **Clinicophysiologic correlations and surgery**	**1940s to 1970s**
• **Infant era**	**mid 1970s to 1990**
• **Developmental era**	**1990 +**

Themes in the 4 eras of pediatric cardiology. As an academic discipline, pediatric cardiology is quite young. Study of the developing embryonic heart has a long history, and pediatric cardiology has always been there, waiting to be discovered and named. The half century from 1936 to the present, the "age of therapy," is still continuing, though we have chosen to subdivide it into three eras.

There is some thematic overlap between the eras shown in Figure 1 and Table 2. Many physiologic concepts were developed during the era of pathologic anatomy, and important new anatopathologic concepts have been added later, during the past fifty years. Nevertheless, thinking in terms of these four eras provides a useful structural background.

Our attempt at a historical review of pediatric cardiology must thus deal with a subject which is rapidly changing in every way, in the state of popular knowledge, in methods of diagnosis and treatment, and in basic concepts. The twentieth century advances in knowledge in the four domains have dramatically changed the prognosis and natural history of heart disease, and have had widespread scientific impact.

Some changes have affected people in their daily lives. Many women, mostly now grandmothers, can remember when the only method of monitoring early heart development was by use of a fetal stethoscope. Now almost all mothers in the Western world have had an ultrasound study, and have seen the beating fetal heart. Thus some knowledge of the **developing heart**, however brief and transient, is today part of common experience, a shared and special joy unknown to previous generations.

Although the anatomy and physiology of the **normal heart** and circulation had been extensively studied by the early twentieth century, there was little recognition of any differences between the hearts of children and adults. With the dawn of the therapeutic era and the beginning of widespread use of cardiac catheterisation in the 1940s and 50s, much new knowledge was gained of the developing heart of childhood, both normal and abnormal.

No doubt medical historians of the future will find much to study in the changing cardiac perspectives of the 20th century. We are too close to the time and to the changes to do more than give an overview. A great deal of the book will, of necessity, deal with changes in the management of **heart defects and childhood heart disease,** since some of these changes are dramatic and within our own experience. However, pediatric cardiology is not confined to the malformed heart, but is a much broader and more challenging field.

Daily life has also been affected by the recognition that some forms of adult heart disease, such as hypertension and atherosclerosis, have their beginnings in childhood. Common wisdom for centuries has advocated exercise and moderation in eating as prescriptions for future health. However, only in this century have careful parents monitored the child's intake of fat and salt, encouraged exercise as not only good in itself but as a preventive of later heart disease. Indeed, parents have sometimes been overwhelmed by a bombardment of information and advice. These parents recognise that keeping a healthy heart is a life long project, and accept the concept, also new in this century, of **preventive cardiology**.

The Pioneers of modern pediatric cardiology are passing into history. They include surgeons, pathologists, men and women from many different scientific backgrounds, and pioneering patients and families. Three pediatric cardiologists had a particularly wide influence on the developing heart of pediatric cardiology. They are Helen Taussig of Baltimore, Alexander Nadas of Boston, and John Keith of Toronto. One of them, Alex Nadas, has recently joined Richard Bing, himself one of the renowned pioneers of cardiac catheterisation, in writing an illuminating overview of the growth of pediatric cardiology [4].

Each of the three started from a pediatric background, and was essentially a self taught cardiologist, and each brought different strengths and vision to the field. The late Richard Rowe, more peripatetic than these three, will always be remembered for his emphasis and skill with infant cardiology, whether working in Auckland New Zealand, in Toronto with John Keith and Peter Vlad, or in Baltimore. In other countries major early contributions were made not only by cardiologists with a pediatric background, but by others specialising in such diverse fields as internal medicine, pathology, and physiology. Two of these many contributions include clarification of the once contentious field of auscultation, and attention to the special problems of the adult born with a heart defect.

History of the four eras. This book is not intended as a biography, or an assessment of individual achievement, but rather an approach to how tools and concepts were used by the pioneers and others to advance knowledge. Pediatric cardiology would not exist as a discipline without the extraordinary work and vision of others in many fields, including surgeons, physiologists, pathologists, nurses, and those in critical care.

A number of excellent historic reviews are available of the history of the circulation [5-6]. Many papers and chapters which illuminated cardiac defects and their management have been reproduced in a readily accessible form [7-9]. The outstanding Classics in Cardiology series has made the work of Peacock and many other early writers available[10]. Bruce Fye has illumined the progress of knowledge of electrocardiography [11], and how this progress has affected both thinking and practice in cardiology. Historic advances in cardiac surgery [12,13], and diagnostic techniques have been well chronicled [14-16]. In preparing this text, it is notable that cardiac surgeons are much more prone than their pediatric colleagues to write with a historical perspective!

Accepting the concept that pediatric cardiology has four domains, the pioneers thus include those who defined the normal heart and circulation, the early embryologists, in addition to those who first described a specific defect or evolved a new treatment. Using this definition the historic approach could become unmanageable, the net too wide to catch a single vision. Yet we have felt it important to acknowledge the breadth of the subject, not reducing the theme to a listing of dates and eponyms, fascinating though these often are. The names of the pioneers, when we know them, are valuable and to be honored; in this text we emphasise the concepts of the pioneers, and how they used the tools they had available in new and sometimes revolutionary ways.

Men, Women, and Ideas. Two of the greatest pioneers, Maude Abbott and Helen Taussig, were women. The role of women in pediatric cardiology may one day be a subject of scholarly study. Prior to the late 19th century the scientific role of women in cardiology was very small, as suggested by the title of that magnificent compilation Circulation of the Blood: Men and Ideas [5]. After the universal recognition of

Maude Abbott as the world's leading expert on the malformed heart [17], women began to emerge from the scientific shadows. Taussig's fame equalled that of her collaborating surgeon, Blalock, and with the publication of her textbook in 1947 [18], she began the definition of congenital malformations of the heart as we think of them today.

From the time of the first Blalock Taussig operation in the mid 1940s, a complex of motives drew women into the new field of therapy. By the early 1940s women formed about 15% of all medical school graduates in the USA, and on graduation a disproportionate number chose the nurturing field of pediatrics as their own. Virtually none had become Department heads, and Taussig's position as a Division chief was rare in the USA and elsewhere.

As one looks back over the past half century, it is possible to recognise that women played a significant role in pediatric cardiology as investigators, in the development of new patterns of cardiac care and teaching, and in other areas including nursing, preventive cardiology, anesthesia and psychosocial studies. Only a few of the pioneers, both men and women, who have formed an integral part of progress in the past extraordinary half century will be named in subsequent chapters.

The Interaction of Tools and Concepts is a difficult but fascinating theme in the history of any scientific endeavor. For example, as Fye has discussed in his history of the electrocardiogram [11], clinicians could recognise an irregular heart beat from the pulse many centuries before Einthoven, yet any systematic approach to rhythm disturbances awaited the tool of the electrocardiogram. In pediatric cardiology concepts of how the heart grows and changes with age have become richer and more complex as new tools of study have developed. The work of all the pioneers was conceptual, but was also influenced by the scientific tools they had available. A major focus here is on how tools and concepts interacted, a focus which supplements the more usual approach of listing major discoverers and some of their accomplishments.

The revolutionary impact of the echocardiogram, a still evolving tool, has affected mainly diagnosis and management. Now that cardiac anatomy and physiology can be imaged with exquisite precision, and the images played back repeatedly far from the actual child, it becomes more of a challenge than in the past to concentrate on the heart in the context of the whole child and family.

The Child with Heart Disease and the interaction of the disease or defect on his family must form part of the history of pediatric cardiology. Medical history in the past has dealt almost entirely with scientific discoveries and personalities. Recently the history of the patients own thoughts and concepts have come under study. Children and patients are also pioneers, and their history has been too little recorded. A child born in 1940 with tetralogy of Fallot, who had a Blalock Taussig anastomosis in 1947 and open repair in 1960, was a pioneer; he and his family faced courageously the hazardous "learning curve" of both new operations before that term was coined.

The child with heart disease through the ages is an elusive topic of study. Some early 18th century writers give a vivid description of the living child, [4,7,8] but such descriptions were rare in the era of pathologic anatomy. In the early part of the therapeutic era, the time of clinicophysiologic correlations and surgery, there was much emphasis on the typical clinical profile, useful in diagnosis, but less on the child in the context of the family and society. Even today, there remains an extraordinary disparity between the volume of medical literature devoted to technical advances, and that devoted to the quality of life of the affected child.

Throughout the text we have attempted to include a few thoughts and writings on childhood, in an effort to reemphasise the theme of the heart and the child.

The Developing Heart: in the first seven chapters of this book we review briefly how the four domains of developmental cardiology, the normal and abnormal heart, and preventive cardiology changed and grew during the different eras. We analyse in some detail the history of 3 specific defects, tetralogy, ventricular septal defect, and double inlet ventricle, and give a brief overview of the growth of pediatric cardiology as an international discipline.

In the final section we include a discussion of current scientific approaches to the developing heart. We also consider a few of the implications of present knowledge, including ethical and quality of life issues and some of the challenges anticipated in the 21st century.

Pediatric cardiology has implications for the child and family, for society in developed and developing countries, and for future biologic research. As long as there are children, the history of pediatric cardiology will continue. This book is written in tribute to the pioneers, some of whom, patients, families, cardiologists and surgeons, we have been fortunate enough to know, admire and love.

REFERENCES AND NOTES

1. Harvey W. Exercitatio anatomica de motu cordis et sanguinis in animalibus, with an English translation by CD Leake. 2nd ed. Springfield Ill: Thomas, 1941.
2. Abbott ME. Atlas of congenital cardiac disease. New York: American Heart Asociation, 1936.
3. Richardson D. A history of the morbus caerulus. Bull Hist Med 1962;36:193-219.
4. Nadas A, Bing RJ. Congenital heart disease. In: Bing RJ, editor. Cardiology: The evolution of the science and the art. Philadelphia: Harwood Academic, 1992: 87-108. Contains photographs of many cardiac pioneers.
5. Fishman AP, Richards DW editors. Circulation of the blood: Men and ideas. New York: Oxford University Press, 1964.
6. Gorny P. Histoire Illustre de la Cardiologie de la Prehistoire a nos jours. Paris: Les Editions Roger Dacosta, 1985.
7. Rashkind WJ. Congenital Heart Disease: Benchmark Papers in Human Physiology/16. Stroudsburg Pa: Hutchinson Ross, 1982. Reproduces a number of important papers, with annotations.
8. Willius FA, Keys TE. Cardiac Classics. A Collection of Classic Works on the Heart and Circulation with Comprehensive Biographic Accounts of the Authors. 2 vols. St Louis: CV Mosby Company, 1941. Reprinted Malabar FL Robert E Krieger 1983,1989.
9. Callahan JA, McGoon DC, Key JD. Classics of Cardiology volume IV (2 parts). Malabar FL: Robert E Krieger, 1989.
10. Peacock TB. On Some of the Causes and Effects of Valvular Disease of the Heart together with On the Prognosis in Cases of Valvular Disease of the Heart. London: John Churchill 1865. Reprinted in Fye WB, ed. Birmingham: The Classics of Cardiology Library, 1990.
11. Fye WB. A history of the origin, evolution and impact of electrocardiography. Am J Cardiol 1994;73:937-949.
12. Shumacker HB Jr. The evolution of cardiac surgery. Bloomington: Indiana University Press, 1992.
13. Johnson SL. The History of Cardiac Surgery 1896-1955. Baltimore: Johns Hopkins University Press 1970.
14. Snellen HA, Dunning AJ, Arntzenius AC, editors. History and perspectives of cardiology: catheterisation, angiocardiography, surgery and concepts of cardiovascular control. Proceedings of meeting Leiden University Nov 1-3 1979. The Hague: Martinius Nijhoff, 1981.
15. Tynan M. Pediatric cardiology: then and now. Cardiology in the Young 1991;1:3-10.
16. Baim D, Bing RJ. Cardiac catheterisation. In: Bing RJ, editor. Cardiology: The evolution of the science and the art. Philadelphia: Harwood Academic, 1992: 1-28.
17. Waugh D. Maudie of McGill: Dr Maude Abbott and the foundation of heart surgery. Toronto: Hannah Institute and Durdrum Press, 1992.
18. Taussig HB. Congenital malformations of the heart. New York Commonwealth Fund 1947. 2nd ed. Cambridge, Harvard University Press for Commonwealth Fund 1960.

CHAPTER 1

Prior To William Harvey

- Growth of knowledge and the two circulations
- Aristotle and the embryonic heart
- Preventive cardiology [?]
- The child with heart disease

"This is the circulation which the blood traverses within us. It has been observed in our time, and will serve to revolutionise all of medicine, just as the invention of the telescope has done for astronomy, the compass has done for commerce, and artillery has done for the whole military art."
Raffaello Magiotti 1637 in a letter to his friends, including Galileo.
Quoted by Bylebyl, J.J., in William Harvey; a conventional medical revolutionary JAMA 239, 1295-1298, 1978.

The Normal Heart and Circulation

The heart and the course of circulation were studied in many lands, over many centuries since the earliest beginnings of scientific enquiry[5,19,20]. The publication of De Motu Cordis[1] by William Harvey in 1628 is one of the major landmarks in the history of medicine. The implications for pediatric cardiology, a discipline yet to be born, were profound, since the nature and relationship of the two circulations, systemic and pulmonary, were now defined.

Magiotti's letter, quoted above, is a striking tribute to the seminal nature of Harvey's discovery. It is also of interest, in the context of our theme of the interaction of tools and concepts, that Magiotti compares the new physiologic "observation" of the circulation with the discovery of new tools namely the telescope, the compass and artillery. Harvey's discovery was not related to any new technology, but rather by the brilliant yet painstaking application of tools already available, he developed a revolutionary and unifying concept.

PRIOR TO WILLIAM HARVEY

In the centuries prior to William Harvey, many writers and artists studied the heart and circulation. In his annotated anthology on the History of Congenital Heart Disease [7] Rashkind reproduced an illustration of a fresco from the cave of Pindal in northern Spain, showing the heart outlined on the surface of a mammoth. He used this to demonstrate that the importance of the heart and its normal position in the left thorax was known to both hunters and artists some 20,000 years ago.

Much of normal cardiac anatomy was well defined by Galen's time, though physiologic concepts of the circulation remained confused for many centuries. Many early writers described the atria as extensions of the veins, rather than integral to the heart, which they believed was composed only of the two ventricles. Recent scholarship has shown that almost all Greek anatomic studies were performed in animals, and that human dissection was shunned. Nevertheless, there was knowledge of the position and anatomic relationships of the heart. Cournand, in reviewing the history of "Air and Blood," [21] quotes from a Hippocratic document "On the Heart" from the 4th century B.C. ascribed to Philiston of Locroi: "The heart is a powerful muscle ... with two distinct ventricles ... The left ventricle is located beneath the right exactly behind the left nipple where its beat can be felt ..." Despite their great anatomic accuracy, the Greek school did not recognise the relation of the pulse to the heart beat, a correlation well known in Egypt in the seventeenth and eighteenth centuries BC, according to the Smith papyrus.

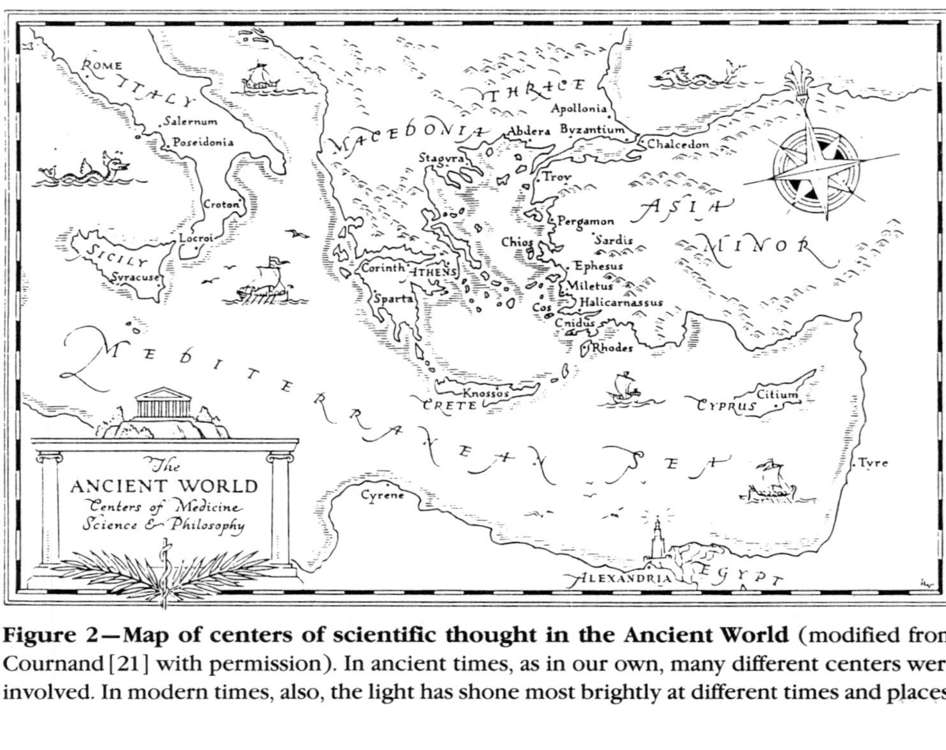

Figure 2—Map of centers of scientific thought in the Ancient World (modified from Cournand [21] with permission). In ancient times, as in our own, many different centers were involved. In modern times, also, the light has shone most brightly at different times and places.

Galen of Pergamon, in the 2nd century AD, performed extensive animal dissections, and also served as physician to the gladiators. He taught that blood passed to the lung, from which waste products were expired, and also that blood and pneuma mixed in the cavity of the left ventricle and were elaborated there into the vital spirit. Pneuma reached the left ventricle through invisible pores in the ventricular septum. Among his many other remarkable observations, Galen defined the phrenic nerve supply of the diaphragm, an anatomic detail that became of great interest to pediatric cardiologists many centuries later, when surgical trauma to the phrenic nerve was a rare and sometimes perplexing cause of postoperative morbidity. He wrote extensively on the pulse, and recounts being able to diagnose that a young girl was in love, rather than ailing, by palpating her "turbulent pulse" when the name of the young man, Pylades, was mentioned. He clearly enjoyed, as later cardiologists have done, the pleasures of being first with a diagnosis.

After the fall of the Roman empire, most Greek writing was lost to the Western world. In the eleventh and twelfth centuries, Galenic teachings were brought to Spain in Arabic translation, together with some new information from Arab medicine. Ibn Nafis, an Arab physician born in Damascus in 1210, claimed that blood mixed with air in the lungs, and also denied the Galenic teaching of invisible pores in the ventricular septum. Michael Servetus (1511-1553) is credited with being the first Westerner to question part of Galen's doctrine. In one chapter in his book "Christianismi Restitutio" he described the passage of blood to the lungs "where it changes color." He also said there are no pores or openings in the ventricular septum. Cournand [21] describes Servetus' life as lonely, and "in almost continuous flight." He was burned at the stake in Geneva for heresy in 1553, a copy of his book attached to his arm. His text was lost for almost a century, but recovered in 1694. Cournand quotes the conclusion reached by Servetus, "He who really understands what is involved in the breathing of man has already sensed the breath of God and thereby saved his soul."

New information on the circulation was added when Fabricius discovered the venous valves, and by the detailed anatomic dissections and drawings of Vesalius in the 16th century. Vesalius, who has been described as the foremost pioneer of modern anatomy, studied in Paris, Pisa, Bologna and Padua before settling in Brussels. It was while he was studying in Padua that he began to separate from Galenic tradition, by basing much of his work on human dissection. [22] Padua thus had an important influence on the lives of both Vesalius and Harvey.

WILLIAM HARVEY

Bylebyl [19] has analysed some of the conceptual and practical hurdles that Harvey needed to overcome before developing the concept published in his monograph "De Motu Cordis" in 1628. Although he was skilled in the dissection of living animals, Harvey said that at first "I could not rightly distinguish how systole and diastole came about ... This was because of the rapidity of the movement ..." He was also hampered by the concept that the blood has certain inherent powers of movement, a concept transmitted from the classic Greek thought. He came to recognise that when the heart contracted blood was expelled into the body from the left ventricle and into the lungs from the right ventricle. But according to Bylebyl's analysis of Harvey's writings,[19] it was not until many years later that by a remarkable and innovative piece of "quantitative reasoning," he came to realise that blood leaving the heart must return to it. "It has been demonstrated that a perpetual movement of blood in a circle is caused by the beat of the heart."[1]

The tools available to Harvey at the time were the relatively simple ones of dissection and ligature also used by his predecessors and contemporaries. His combination of tireless experiment with deductive reasoning led him to the illumination of a previously dark and confusing field of science. As Bylebyl and others have noted however, although Harvey's new theory was immediately embraced by scientists, it caused little if any change in medical practice. Blood letting and other empiric approaches were scarcely influenced, perhaps not least because no other treatments were available.

The Developing Heart

The beginnings of the heart beat aroused interest from early times. Needham[23] describes how Aristotle, in the 4th cent B.C., observed the embryonic chick heart beating at various stages and declared "The heart is the principle and origin of the embryo." Needham illustrates on an ingenious chart the history of embryology from 600 B.C. to 600 A.D., together with the contemporary events and persons. He mentions that Galen, who did most of his writing between A.D. 150 and 180, wrote less than one of his twenty collected volumes on the subject of embryology. Needham quotes Galen as dividing the effects of the "faculties" or natural entities into three, genesis, growth and nutrition.

> *"Genesis (or embryogenesis) is not a simple activity of Nature, but is compounded of alteration and of shaping ... in order that the substance may acquire its appropriate shape and position, its cavities, outgrowths and attachments, and so forth, it has to undergo a shaping or formative process. One would be justified in calling this substance which undergoes alteration the material of an animal, just as wood is the material of a ship and wax of an image."*

Needham describes this as "a very remarkable passage," suggesting some quite modern views about growth and differentiation. Even today, as we enter the developmental era, we are obliged to agree with Galen that genesis, including the embryonic growth of the heart, is not a simple matter.

Detailed systematic study of the developing heart awaited the discovery of the microscope, many centuries later. Leonardo da Vinci's exquisite drawings of the embryo are now widely known, but only became available to the public when they were reproduced in the late nineteenth century. Needham reproduces some of Leonardo's illustrations, and quotes many scientists and writers, including Dante, who studied or wrote on embryonic growth.

THE DUCTUS ARTERIOSUS AND FORAMEN OVALE

Galen knew of both of these structures, and their normal closure after birth. Geoffrey Dawes, himself a remarkable pioneer in perinatal physiology, has written of the growth of knowledge of the newborn heart. [21a] He credits Fabricius, an anatomist and embryologist writing in the the early 1600s, with being the first to illustrate these patent fetal channels in the lamb and the human fetus, and showing the inferior vena cava directed towards the foramen ovale.

Cardiac Defects and Childhood Heart Disease

Although heart abnormalities were ocasionally reported, childhood heart disease was not a subject of scientific study in the centuries prior to William Harvey. Knowledge of the normal heart and circulation was gradually accumulating, but differentiation of cardiac disorders from other maladies proved a difficult task.

Rashkind [7] states "exactly when physicians recognised heart disease is difficult to pinpoint ... and even more difficult to determine when they first became aware of congenital heart disease." He reproduced a Babylonian tablet, dating from at least 2,000 B.C., with the inscription "When a woman gives birth to an infant that has the heart open and has no skin, the country will suffer from calamities." Rashkind proposed this as the first description of ectopia cordis, while acknowledging some argument regarding the translation.

Galen is generally recognised as describing the anatomy of the foramen ovale and ductus arteriosus, and their normal closure after birth. Rashkind has attributed to Leonardo da Vinci the first drawing of an atrial septal defect. [24] He noted that Leonardo described and illustrated this in 1513 in his Quarderni d'Anatomia, saying "I have found from a, left auricle to b, right auricle, a perforating channel from a to b which I note here to see whether this occurs in other auricles of other hearts." According to Rashkind, 130 years elapsed before another such observation was made. Gassendi in 1640 reported a patent foramen ovale in an adult female.

RECOGNITION OF HEART DISEASE

Attempts to define and categorise heart problems in either children or adults are not recorded prior to Harvey's discovery of the normal circulation. Abelmann and his colleagues, [25] in a scholarly discussion of the early history of myocardial failure, describe some of the difficulties encountered by clinicians. First, the role of the heart as a pump was not yet accepted, and second, many symptoms involved other organs such as the lungs and liver. When symptoms of systemic or pulmonary congestion were accompanied by irregularities of the pulse, heart disease was sometimes suspected. Some symptoms of heart failure, including dyspnea and pulmonary edema, were described in adults by Avicenna as early as the 11th century, but clear attribution of such symptoms to the heart was first made by Marcello Malpighi later in the 17th century. [25] Abelman quotes a vivid description by Carolus Piso in 1618 of paroxysmal nocturnal dyspnea in an octogenarian, but there seems to have been no recognition of such symptoms in infancy prior to the 20th century.

Rashkind [24] reproduced some early paintings of adults with a bluish tinge to their skin, which he used in illustrating his ebullient lectures on history. It is difficult, centuries later, to be sure if these paintings represented artistic license, peripheral cyanosis, or true pioneering observations. So far as we know, the first accounts of the symptoms of a cyanotic child did not occur till the 18th century.

Preventive Cardiology

Cardiology was not yet envisioned as a specialty, and it is not surprising that risk factors for adult heart disease attracted little attention. Gotto [26] quotes Leonardo da Vinci, commenting on his drawing, The Anatomy of the Old Man: "Vessels in the elderly, through the thickenings of the tunics, restrict the transit of the blood." Any concept of the prevention of such thickening of the tunics lay far in the future.

However, two activities now recommended by various Task Forces on heart health were discussed even before Harvey's time, namely avoidance of tobacco and regular exercise. Tobacco was imported to Europe from the New World early in the 17th century, and became, as it has remained, a substance of impassioned argument. It certainly was not generally recognised as being toxic to the heart or lungs. Indeed Harley, [27] in a fascinating history of tobacco, describes how some physicians actually prescribed it for asthma and breast disease, while Giles Verard of Antwerp in 1587 called it a panacea curing all ills. However, tobacco had some distinguished opponents. Harley also recounts that Ben Jonson in "Every Man in his Humor" has Cob say "Its good for nothing but to choake a man, and fill him full of smoake and imbers." According to Harley, King James I of England was strongly against tobacco on moral grounds, but also said "The generall good liking and imbracing of this foolish custom doeth but onely proceede from that affectation of noueltie, and popular error." In these days of open season on monarchial thoughts, it is refreshing to acknowledge both King James I and "rare" Ben Jonson as unwitting pioneers in preventive cardiology! Harley also quotes the playright Beaumont, centuries before jogging, as asking,

... "should we not take some wholesome exercise
To chafe our vaines, and stretch our arteries ..."

The Child with Heart Disease

At present, the child with heart disease in the ages prior to Harvey remains a very elusive figure. Historians of the future may be able to give more details, as more attention is paid to documents dealing with daily life in the past. Infant mortality was high from many causes, and it is likely that the possibility of cardiac disease as a cause of death was not even considered.

Some deforming extracardiac congenital abnormalities were recognised clinically from early times. Vesalius described both the symptoms and the anatomic findings in a two year old girl with hydrocephalus, referring to "that ailment the ancients call hydrocephalus." [22a]

There is an increasing interest among medical historians in the history of the sick. Porter [28,29] maintains that although the history of the sick cannot be written in the same sequential way as the chronicle of medicine and of doctors, "that does not mean it cannot or should not be written at all." He describes some of the interactions between physicians and their self-medicating adult patients in England in the 17th and 18th centuries. He quotes a certain Margaret Paston in 1464 as counselling a friend, *"For Goddys sake be war what medesyns ye take of any fysissyans of London."* Although there are a number of accounts by diarists and letter writers of their own symptoms and attempts at treatment, detailed lay accounts of childhood health problems from early centuries seem almost non-existent. It is possible this lack is due to some degree of fatalism in the centuries of high infant and child mortality. Porter comments that when there were no effective medical treatments, lay people and physicians alike set great store by the Hippocratic concept that it was each individual's duty to regulate his own health and maintain a healthy life style. Despite the lack of early writing, we support Porter's contention that patients are not "in some sense 'subhistorical,' timeless objects merely waiting to be treated by doctors who are part of progress."

Linda Pollock, [30] in a study of parents writing about their children prior to the 20th century, mentions that letters and diaries often show evidence of "searing grief" when a child was seriously ill or died. She disagrees vehemently with the view often expressed by others that childhood loss, being frequent in prior centuries, was almost a matter of indifference. She states that despite all the recent work on the history of childhood, "we still know little of actual childhood."

The history of all areas of medicine will be enriched as more is learned of the lives of children of the past, both in sickness and in health (Figure 3).

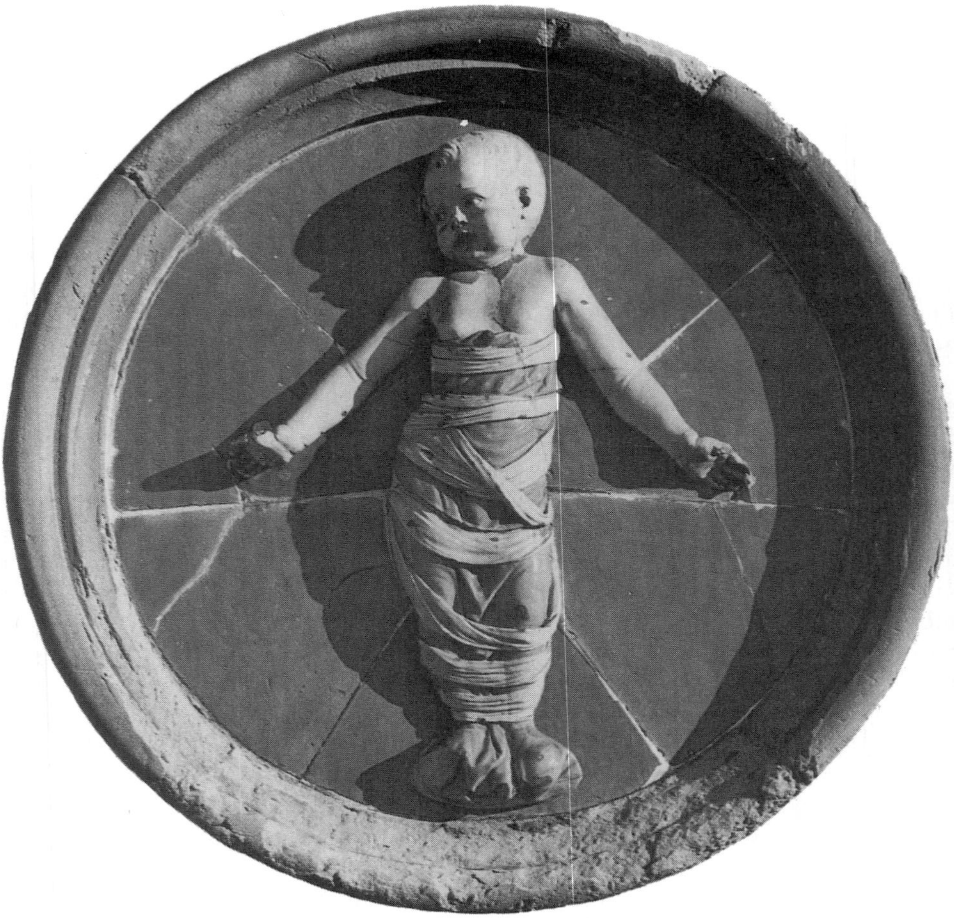

Figure 3—The infant: The terra cotta infants of Della Robbia, from the Ospedale degli Innocenti in Florence c.1463, remind us of the mystery of childhood in past centuries.

ADDITIONAL REFERENCES AND NOTES

19. Bylebyl JJ. William Harvey, a conventional medical revolutionary JAMA 1978;239: 1295-1298.

20. Bing RJ. Cardiology. The evolution of the science and the art. Philadelphia: Harwood Academic Publishers, 1992.

21. Cournand A. Air and blood. In: Fishman AP, Richards DW editors. Circulation of the blood. Men and ideas. New York: Oxford University Press 1964: 3-70

21a. Dawes GS. Physiologic changes in the circulation at birth. In: ibid 1982:743-815.

22. O'Malley CD: Andreas Vesalius of Brussels 1514-1564. Berkely and Los Angeles: Univ. of Californa Press, 1964.

22a Ibid p.253.

23. Needham J. Embryology in antiquity. In: A History of Embryology.Needham J, Hughes A editors. 2nd ed. New York: Abelard-Schuman, 1959:18-74.

24. Rashkind WJ. Historic aspects of congenital heart disease. Birth Defects Original Article Series. Baltimore, Williams and Wilkins for National Foundation, 1972;8:2-8.

25. Abelmann W, Katz AM, Bing RJ: Myocardial failure: Early history, biochemistry, receptors and contractile proteins. In: Bing RJ editor. Cardiology. The evolution of the science and the art. Philadelphia: Harwood Academic Publishers, 1992: 201-227.

26. Gotto AM Jr. Some reflections on arteriosclerosis: past, present and future. Circulation 1985;72:8-17.

27. Harley D. The beginnings of the tobacco controversy: puritanism, James I, and the royal physicians. Bull Hist Med 1993;67:28-50.

28. Porter R: The patient's view. Doing medical history from below. Theory and Society. 1985;14:175-198.

29. Porter R: The patient in England, c. 1660-c.1800. In: Medicine in Society. Wear A. editor. Cambridge: Cambridge Univ. Press 1992: 91-105.

30. Pollock LA. Forgotten Children. Parent-child relations from 1500 to 1900. Cambridge Univ. Press, 1983:125-140.

CHAPTER 2

From Harvey to the mid 19th century

- The 2 centuries from Harvey to Peacock
- Pathologic anatomy of specific defects
- New tools, the microscope, sphygmomanometer, stethoscope
- Concepts of blood pressure, cyanosis, murmurs
- Early descriptions of how heart problems affect the child

Introduction

A period of 230 years separated the publication of William Harvey's De Motu Cordis from the appearance of Thomas Peacock's treatise on Malformations of the Human Heart. [31] Many important changes occurred in thinking about the heart during these two centuries, a time period which can be thought of in the history of pediatric cardiology as the age from Harvey to Peacock.

Although pathologic anatomy was still dominant, physiologic concepts were continually evolving, aided by new tools allowing for measurement and documentation of concepts previously based on theory or anatomic observation alone.

The Normal Heart and Circulation

Harvey's discovery had provided a great impetus to further studies of the normal heart and circulation. The capillary circulation was first demonstrated in the lungs of frogs by Marcello Malpighi of Bologna only thirty three years after Harvey's monograph. As the tools available became more powerful and sophisticated, lenses and microscopes were increasingly used in study of the circulation. Table 3 shows a few of the physiologic concepts emerging during this era of pathologic anatomy.

Table 3
PHYSIOLOGIC CONCEPTS IN THE PATHOLOGIC ANATOMY ERA

Year	Concept	Tools
1628	Harvey normal circulation, disappearance of Galen's 'invisible pores' [1,19]	pathologic experiment
1669	Lower uptake of 'air' in lungs [21]	animal studies
1733	Hales blood pressure in horse [5]	arterial cannula
1779	Lavoisier 'air in lung to red color blood' [21]	
1797	Baillie 'livid color' in transposition ? first clinicopathologic correlation [7]	
1819	Laennec [32]	stethoscope
1828	Poiseuille human blood pressure	mercury manometer
1858	Peacock localisation of murmur [31]	

A number of the original papers describing early discoveries began to be collected and duplicated by Willius and Keys in 1941, [8] and this valuable work has since been continued and amplified. [9]

By the middle of the 19th century, the concept of systemic blood pressure was now a measurable phenomenon, though the tools of measurement were unwieldy, and the value to be derived from such measurements by the clinician was still far from clear. Oxygen was now known to be the component of air which led to the normal change in color of blood as it traversed the lungs. [21]

THE MURMURING HEART

Laennec's invention of the monaural wooden stethoscope did not immediately convert all physicians into ardent auscultators, but it greatly extended the ability of the physician to develop clinicophysiologic concepts applicable at the bedside. The stethoscope was used for diagnosis of both heart and lung disease, though separation of the two remained a source of difficulty.

Even by the early nineteenth century, abnormalities of the heart valves, including mitral and aortic stenosis, were recognised by cardiac pathologists and clinicians interested in the heart. The stethoscope was thus at first used primarily in the diagnosis of valvar disease. Peacock [31] stated that in older patients with pulmonic stenosis, a "*loud systolic murmur will be heard ... audible very distinctly in the course of the pulmonary artery, or from the base of the heart towards the middle of the left clavicle...*" Thus, by the time Peacock wrote, [31a] it was beginning to be recognised that auscultation could have localising value in both heart and lung disease. At first clinicophysiolologic correlations were based only on comparing auscultatory with autopsy findings. But Peacock's phraseology on murmur transmission suggests that even 140 years ago the finest physicians were seeking to link cardiac physiology with anatomy, and structural anomalies with function.

ELECTRICITY AND PHYSIOLOGY

There was no single flash of insight during these two centuries comparable to Harvey's discovery of the circulation, but a series of new ways of measuring natural phenomena were laying the groundwork for cardiac physiology in the future. Many discoveries of import for the future of cardiology were made during this period. We will cite but two examples, the experiments of Galvani, and Steno's concept of the heart as muscle, an essential concept before myocardial research could begin.

Luigi Galvani of Bologna, a Professor of anatomy who also practiced obstetrics, had a particular interest in electricity. His experiments, as Hellerstein remarks in a brilliantly readable account, [33] are "now listed in the annals of history." Galvani's observation in 1756 that an electrical current could cause twitching in the leg muscles of a frog led him to the concept of electricity as an important physiologic phenomenon. This insight, followed by many subsequent experiments, disagreements with Volta, and gradually improving technology preceded the work of Einthoven by about 150 years. Einthoven's development of the electrocardiogram in the early years of the 20th century, later became important to pediatric cardiologists when they began to appear in the 1940s, to their patients, and to the flourishing modern field of electrophysiology.

HEART MUSCLE

Stensen, also known as Steno, is described by Nadas and Bing, [4] in their outline of the life of this Danish physician, as "one of the least known but brilliant and imaginative scientists of the Baroque era." He wrote extensively on anatomy, saying of the heart *"Some have greeted the heart as the sun, others as the king: but if you examine it more closely, one finds it to be nothing more than muscle."* This observation of the muscular structure of the heart aroused controversy, but led to later recognition by von Haller and by Albertini, [25] that heart failure might be due to weakening of cardiac muscle, conceptualised even later as "pump failure."

The Developing Heart

A number of theories began to be elaborated on the differences between embryonic mammalian hearts and those of more primitive organisms. The microscope allowed much more intensive and detailed study of the embryonic heart than was possible in earlier centuries.

Peacock, [31] among his many contributions to the study of childhood heart disease, was also interested in etiology, or risk factors for cardiac defects. He comments:

"In the production of defective development, sex has been supposed to exercise an influence, and malformations are certainly most common in males, though why

it should be so seems incapable of explanation. I find however, that of ninety-one cases of malformation which I have collected, and in which the sex of the subjects is recorded, fifty two were males, and thirty nine females, or 57.2% and 42.8% respectively." He remarks in another passage *"In other instances, also, there has apparently been an hereditary predisposition to defective development of the heart, more than one child of the same parents having been affected."*

Later historians will probably find earlier refences to suspected genetic influences on cardiac growth, but Peacock was clearly applying some epidemiologic concepts to his meticulous collection of pathologic and clinical observations. His words presage the long period of collection of data on genetic and familial aspects of heart malformations, a process which continues using vastly more sophisticated tools, to the present day.

The passionate interest of parents in the etiology of heart defects was first mentioned by Steno (Figure 4), writing in Copenhagen in 1673.

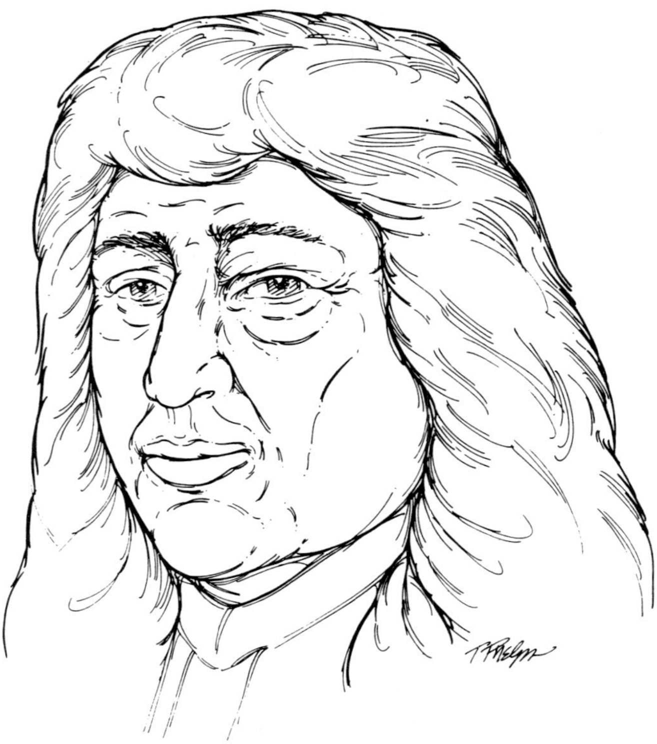

Figure 4—Steno. Niels Stensen (1638-1686), Danish physician and anatomist.

Cardiac Defects and Childhood Heart Disease

During this era the tools of the pathologist led to growing understanding of the anatomic details of the normal heart. A number of case reports on cardiac defects began to appear, sometimes combined with a history of the child's symptoms during life.

Specific cardiac malformations began to arouse interest, and some were described in detail. [4,7,10,34,35] Stensen, also known as Steno, published in 1673 [36] what is now credited with being the first anatomic description of tetralogy of Fallot, [4,7,37] a description discussed in more detail in chapter 7. The stillborn infant had multiple additional defects, including bifid sternum and omphalocele, syndactyly, and cleft lip and palate.

Sandifort in 1777 [38] described the anatomic findings in a child with tetralogy of Fallot, calling this a "very rare disease of the heart." The chapter containing this historic account has been reproduced in full and analysed by Bennet. [39] Sandifort, who called the child a "Blue Boy," mentioned that he was a clever boy, becoming perhaps the first author to document that persistent cyanosis is not in and of itself a cause of mental retardation. He described the blue color of the fingers and the "sinking spells" which had begun after one year of age. He commented that at autopsy the aorta was "springing from both ventricles, and had to receive all the blood from both." Nadas and Bing [4] give an account of Sandifort's life, and quote his introduction to the autopsy findings:

> *"How great was the surprise of the onlookers, how great equally was my own surprise, when we saw the point of the finger to stretch into the aorta, which is not at all accustomed to maintain communications with the right ventricle, in conformity with the otherwise constant laws of nature!"*

In addition to his refreshing candor, and his detailed and meticulous illustrative plates, Sandifort's chapter was distinguished by his review of prior reports, including that of Steno. He mentions that Steno had also found the right ventricle to have three openings, "one from the auricle, two into the arteries, and this same duct of the aorta, common to each ventricle, formed a double orifice in the middle septum of the heart." The term "overriding aorta" had yet to be used, but there is no doubt from his text, or from the illustration showing a probe in the aorta, [39] that this is what Sandifort was describing. His was a pioneering description of symptoms and anatomic findings in the same child.

Before giving his detailed report and literature review, Sandifort opens his chapter with a statement deploring the difficulty of diagnosis and prognosis in "diseases of the chest . . . *They even deceive the most experienced, and the Leaders of Medicine themselves! And not infrequently they carry off the sturdiest men, breathing out health itself, in the midst of strenuous tasks or in the gaiety of conversation, death being very sudden . . ."*

This passage describes in rather moving terms, not only diagnostic frustration, but an awareness of the lurking menace of sudden cardiac death. It also suggests that the interior of the chest was still a mysterious region, and a lack of certainty if sudden death in the "sturdiest men" was of cardiac or pulmonary origin.

William Hunter, about seven years later in 1784, described the cyanotic spells ('fits'), and the growth pattern of a boy with tetralogy who lived to thirteen years of age. [7,40] He reflected on the difference between this boy and an infant decribed in the same paper who had died at thirteen days with anatomic findings of pulmonary atresia and intact ventricular septum:

> *"In the first and second case, the material disadvantage seems to have been, the want of the full effect of respiration on the blood. In the first case, so little of the blood passed through the lungs, that life was extinguished in thirteen days: in the second, enough passed through the lungs to support a weak and tottering life for as many years.*
>
> *As the carnation tint of complexion depends on the florid colour of the blood, the dark or grey complexion of both these patients corresponds particularly with the observation of the latest philosophers, we might say, indeed of all ages, that the blood takes its bright hue in the lungs from respiration ..."*
>
> *Later, analysing the autopsy findings, "the pulmonary artery was as thin in its substance as any common vein: though it was very small at its beginning, yet at a small distance from the heart, it became gradually almost as large as common.*
>
> *From these appearances it was plain that in the living body, 1. A very small quantity only of blood (instead of the whole) passed through the lungs to receive the benefit of respiration, and that with a small force too ..."*

Hunter's comment on the small force of the pulmonary blood flow was very prescient. He gave the opinion, while the child was still alive, that there was "a peculiarity of constitution about the heart ... which we could not suppose that any medicine would reach" and he made an impassioned plea that a knowledge of incurable complaints should restrain us "from bleeding, blistering, vomiting purging, cutting tissues, applying caustics; in a word torturing a miserable and incurable human creature." Farre [41] criticised this statement, saying "it is not enough to refrain from inflicting pain ... we must sooth and mitigate the evil which nature does not, and art cannot cure." It seems likely that patients would have supported Hunter, had they been aware of this controversy!

Hunter clearly attributes the cyanosis to failure of blood to reach the lungs for oxygenation. The concept that the child's cyanosis was due to a right to left shunt, rather than directly to the pulmonic stenosis, remained elusive and controversial for at least another 150 years. [4,42]

Despite the meticulous and pioneering nature of these case reports, they lack some of the extraordinary conceptual vision shown by Baillie, [7,43] who in 1797 was probably the first to use the term "admixture" in the context of complete transposition. He described the cardiac anatomy in a two month old infant with:

> *"a very singular malformation of the heart ... the aorta arose out of the right ventricle, and the pulmonary artery out of the left ... a florid blood must always have been circulating between the lungs and the left side of the heart, except for the admixture of the dark blood which passed through the foramen ovale; and a dark blood must always have been circulating between the right side of the heart and the ... body, except for the very small quantity of florid blood which passed into the aorta by the remains of the ductus arteriosus." He attributed the "most unusually livid color of the skin" to the small proportion of "florid blood" in the general circulation.*

Baillie thus described vividly the modern concept that in the singular malformation later known as transposition, the two circulations are in parallel, rather than in series, as is normal. It was to take 150 years and the development of many new tools and concepts, before any attempt was made to increase intracardiac mixing in complete transposition.

DIGITALIS

The end of the 18th century was remarkable for another discovery, or rediscovery, to have profound effects on cardiology. Although digitalis had been named in 1542, and had been used as an expectorant or emetic since the 13th century, it was not in regular use by physicians until Withering's paper of 1785. [44,44a] Although Withering advised use of the drug mainly as a diuretic, he was aware of its effects on the heart, including slowing of the pulse rate, and was also well aware of its possible toxic effects. He mentions using the drug in only a few children, one of whom, a three year old boy with ascites and anasarca "got perfectly well." Tried as a last resort in a seven year old boy with hydrocephalus, "after three days, no sensible effects taking place, digitalis was omitted and the mercurial plan of treatment adopted."

Withering reportedly faced his own mortality with an admirable wry humor, remarking of himself in his latter days: "The flower of physicians is indeed Withering."

THE DREAM OF DIAGNOSIS

Farre [41] expressed discontent with the contemporary state of cardiac diagnosis in 1814:

> *"The Clinical Physician ... will content himself with saying that his patient labours under some disease of the heart ... But if words would be the sign of ideas, how loose and imperfect must be the conceptions of diseases, which by the very expression, are thus rudely blended and confounded!"*

Farre's moving plea for greater specificity of diagnosis remained long unanswered. The tools available to the early pioneers seeking to correlate clinical and pathologic findings were scanty, but their attention to the clinical history and meticulous regard of anatomic detail is impressive. Seventy four years after Farre wrote of the rude blending and confounding of diagnoses, Fallot [45] made a specific premortem diagnosis in a 36 year old cyanotic man in Marseilles; but it was to be many more years before this singular achievement could be reproduced by others.

Preventive Cardiology

This area of study did not advance greatly during the 2 centuries between Harvey and Peacock. Although Poiseuille had developed a mercury manometer in 1828, a practical method was not in use until the work of Marey in Paris in 1863.

The anatomy of the coronary circulation was well known to William Harvey.

During the late 18th and early 19th century coronary artery disease began to be recognised as a clinical entity, starting with Morgagni's publication of De Sedibus et Causis Morborum in 1761. [46] John Hunter described his own recurrent attacks of angina, William Heberden provided a classic description of angina pectoris, and Alan Burns in 1809 [46] described this condition as being due to reduced coronary blood flow.

Gotto [26] quotes John Fothergill (1712-1780), who advised adoption, after the appearance of symptoms of chest pain, of "a plan of restricted food, which might greatly retard the progress of the disorder, and to restrain excesses of passion and anxiety ..." This advice suggests the concept of secondary prevention, once angina pectoris was present. The concept of primary prevention of atherosclerosis lay 200 years in the future, in the therapeutic age.

The Child with Heart Disease

The abnormal signs and symptoms of a child with cyanotic heart disease are now more clearly presented in the medical literature than in earlier years. Careful medical histories which include descriptions of cyanotic spells and retarded growth were provided by several authors. As new tools were developed, the concept grew that medicine was advancing beyond Farre's "loose and imperfect" diagnosis that his patient "labours under some disease of the heart." The concept was emerging that a specific diagnosis might at times be attainable. The search for a clinicophysiologic profile of disease had begun, but this was as yet far removed from any hope of benefiting the individual child.

Hunter [40] was perhaps the first author to convey movingly the stress of a child's severe heart disease upon the family. Describing his visit to the intensely cyanotic newborn infant later found to have pulmonary atresia with an intact septum, he comments how the nurse signalled that something was very wrong: *"she durst not speak, for fear of alarming the mother."* And again, in his description of the eleven year old boy with tetralogy: *"he had been reared with the utmost attention; and his affectionate parents hardly ever durst entertain hopes of his arriving at the age of manhood ... and I hinted to the father, who despaired of his living at any time, if he should be carried off in one of these fits, that it would be unpardonable to neglect the opportunity of discovering the cause of his ill health."* The parents listened to Hunter's plea, showing a loving care that one day their own and their son's tragedy might indeed help others.

REFERENCES AND NOTES

31. Peacock TB. On Malformations of the Human Heart. London. John Churchill, 1858.

31a. Porter IH. The nineteenth-century physician and cardiologist Thomas Bevill Peacock (1812-82). Medical History 1962;6:240-254.

32. Laennec RTH. Traite de l'auscultation mediate. 2 vols. Paris: J.S.Chaude, 1826.

33. Hellerstein H. Electrophysiology, electrocardiography, cardiopulmonary resuscitation. In: Bing RJ editor. Cardiology: The evolution of the science and the art. Philadelphia: Harwood Academic 1992:255-296.

34. Bouillaud JB. Traite Clinique des Maladies du Coeur. Paris, J.B.Bailliere, 2 vols. 1841.

35. Senac JB. Traite de la Structure du Coeur, de son Action, et de ses Maladies. Paris: Briasson, 1749.

36 Stensen N. Embryo monstro affinis Parisiis dissectus. Acta medica et philosophica Hafniencia 1673;1:202-203. Reprinted in Maar V. editor Stenonis Nicolai:Opera philosophica Copenhagen 1910;2: 49-53.

36a. Warburg E. Niels Steesens Beskrivelse af der forste publicerede Tilfaelde of "Fallot's Tetrade." Nord Med 1942;16:3550-3551.

37. Willius FA. An unusually early description of the so-called tetralogy of Fallot. Proc Staff Meetings Mayo Clinic 1948;23:316-320.

38 Sandifort E. Observationes anatomo-pathologicae. Leyden, P.v.d Eyk and D.Vygh 1777.

39. Bennet LR. Sandifort's "Observationes," Chapter 1, concerning a very rare disease of the heart. I. Tetralogy of Fallot or Sandifort? Bull Hist Med 1946;20:539-570. Bennet reproduces the manuscript (translated into English from the original Latin), and the 3 accompanying plates, and gives an interesting account of Sandifort's life. The original ms had been studied in the Army Medical library, Cleveland branch.

40. Hunter W. Three cases of malformation of the heart in: Medical Observations and Inquiries vol 6, Society of Physicians in London, London: T.Cadell, 1784.

41. Farre JR. Pathological Researches. Essay I. On Malformations of the Human Heart. London: Longman Hurst Rees Orme and Brown, 1814.

42. Bing RJ. The Johns Hopkins: The Blalock-Taussig era. Persp Biol Med 1988;32:85-90.

43. Rodin AE. The influence of Matthew Baillie's Morbid Anatomy: biography, evaluation and reprint. Springfield: Charles C. Thomas, 1973:91-92.

43a. Baillie M. Of a remarkable transposition of the viscera. Philosophic Transactions of the Royal Society 1788;78:350-356.

44. Withering W. An account of the foxglove and some of its medicinal uses: with practical remarks on dropsy and other diseases. Birmingham, M.Swinney 1785.

44a. May LA. Withering on the foxglove and other classics in pharmacology. Oceanside NY, Dabor Science 1977:1-207. contains facsimile of original communication by Withering.

45. Fallot A. Contribution a l'anatomie pathologique de la maladie bleue (cyanose cardiaque). Marseille Medicale 1888: 71-93, 138-158, 207-223, 270-286, 341-354.

46. Paul O, Bing RJ. Coronary artery disease. In: Bing RJ editor. Cardiology: The evolution of the science and the art. Philadelphia, Harwood Academic 1992:145-167.

CHAPTER 3

Late 19th to early 20th century

- From Peacock to Abbott
- New tools, Xray, EKG, fluoroscope
- Clinical profile of specific defects (Roger, Fallot, Abbott)
- Embryologic advances
- The child with heart disease

"The search for the truth is in one way difficult, in another way easy. For it is evident that no one is able to attain it completely, nor to miss it altogether, but each can contribute something to knowledge of nature. From gathering together of all these things there arises a great structure."

—Aristotle in Metaphysics Book A: quoted on National Academy of Sciences building.

Introduction

Cardiac knowledge advanced rapidly in the late 19th and early 20th century,[47] even though this was still the age before therapy, the era of pathologic anatomy. The culmination of this era in the history of pediatric cardiology came with the publication in 1936 of Maude Abbott's great Atlas of congenital cardiac disease.[2]

During the almost eighty years which separated the publication of Peacock's treatise on cardiac malformations[10] from that of Abbott, there was little effective therapy for childhood heart problems. Medications such as digitalis, quinidine, and mercurial diuretics were already in use, though their action and indications were poorly understood. In adults, nitroglycerine had been used for relief of angina pectoris since the early 1880s, and in both children and adults salicylates were given for treatment of acute rheumatic fever. The specialty of pediatrics was in its formative years. Infants and children were subject to many more infectious and respiratory diseases than now. Without many of the tools of modern evaluation, lacking the knowledge of the physiology of tachypnea and pulmonary venous congestion, even the diagnosis of arrhythmia or congestive heart failure in a young child was still a major challenge.

During the era before effective treatment, the tools of the pathologist led to an excellent understanding of the anatomic details of the normal heart, and of almost all known cardiac defects. Experimental physiology was developing into a recognised discipline, and the implications of laboratory studies began to be introduced into clinical thinking. New diagnostic tools, including the chest Xray and electrocardiogram, brought a fresh approach to the heart. These tools began to be used early in the 20th century, as shown diagrammatically in Figure 1.

The eventual impact of these changes in both thinking and technology was momentous, and a new cadre of physicians, later to be known as cardiologists, began to specialise in the study of the heart, and the integration of cardiac knowledge and patient care. In the meantime surgeons were acquiring some experience with thoracic surgery, though approach to the heart itself was still considered treacherous.

The Normal Cardiovascular System

By 1936, the end of the pretherapeutic age, a good deal of the physiology of the normal heart in animals was well understood. Although Pohlman [48,49] and others had written on the fetal circulation and on changes at birth, there seems to have been little study of, or interest in, how the physiology of a normal child might differ from an adult. The concept that infants and children were physiologically distinct from small adults had not yet become part of medical thinking.

This period also saw the development of a clinically useful sphygmomanometer, the first cardiac catheterisations in animals, [16,55,55a] and an exponential growth in knowledge of cardiac receptors and biochemistry. [25] Fye [47] dates the beginning of physiology as a formal discipline in the USA to 1871, when Henry Pickering Bowditch returned from studying with Carl Ludwig in Leipzig and founded the new department of physiology at Harvard. A few years later, in 1876, Newell Martin established a program of advanced research training in physiology at Johns Hopkins, and developed an isolated mammalian heart preparation which was widely used.

A few physiologic concepts with a special importance to pediatric heart disease are shown in Table 4.

Table 4
PHYSIOLOGIC CONCEPTS 1866-1936: THE PEACOCK-ABBOTT DECADES

Year	Concept	Tools
1870	Fick principle [50]	(awaited tool of catheterisation)
1879	Roger specificity of murmur[51]	stethoscope
1888	Fallot cyanosis in tetralogy[45]	clinical history + pathology
1907	Keith and Flack-SA node [52]	physiology, microscopy
1911	Gibson physiology of murmur[53]	
1914	Starling Law [54]	physiology laboratory
1936	Abbott clinicopathologic profile	auscultatory diagram[2] Xray, electrocardiogram

It is part of the fascination of history that silent and extraordinary events are occurring without pomp or fanfare, unnoticed by many experts in the field. Such an event was Werner Forssman's passage of a catheter into his own heart in the summer of 1929. [7,16,56] The story of the tumultuous reception of this experiment has been well told. [7,16] Forssman's chief, Professor Sauerbruch of Berlin reportedly fired him, saying that such work as cardiac catheterisation had no place in a Department of surgery: "For a real surgeon there is only one thing, to operate, to operate, to operate." [16]

There have been many more histories of cardiac catheterisation than of pediatric cardiology. Even after reading some of these histories, it remains mysterious why no cardiac specialist immediately elected to follow up on the now long established animal work, which had shown since 1861 that a catheter could safely be passed into the heart of an animal. Did cardiologists in 1928 believe that with their new tools of Xray, fluoroscopy and 3 lead electrocardiogram, they did not need to think of applying animal work to humans? Was the gulf between laboratory physicians ("physiologists") and clinicians even deeper than it is today? Yet the statements of Gibson and Roger, and no doubt many others unknown to us, indicate that clinicians were eager to apply new physiologic knowledge to their patients.

These rhetorical questions do not tell us why it fell to a young surgeon to pass the first catheter into a human heart-his own. Forssman's original paper is well worth rereading for the stark simplicity of his account of this feat, illustrated by a chest Xray showing the catheter in the right atrium. Possibly at that time in history, only a surgeon, and a young one, accustomed to thinking invasively, could have successfully addressed the three questions underlying all great innovations: Can it be done? Should it be done? Shall I do it? His accomplishment was ultimately honored by the Nobel Prize, awarded in 1956 jointly to Forssman, Andre Cournand and Dickinson Richards. Cournand and Richards began to collaborate at Bellevue Hospital New York in 1932, and transformed cardiac catheterisation in the human from a lonely experiment to a coordinated team approach to cardiopulmonary physiology.

The Developing Heart

As the tools of pathologic dissection, microscopy, and serial sections developed, the early embryologists published a series of exquisite descriptive studies. [49,57-59] They defined in detail the morphologic progression from a muscle wrapped tube to the four-chambered heart. [60] These contributions were later reviewed by van Mierop. [61] In 1914 Mall [62] pioneered the concept of staging embryo development, work later elaborated by Streeter [63] and O'Rahilly. [64] Staging allowed for the graphic depiction of simultaneous growth of the heart and other organs. Experimental embryology began during this period. [65]

Early anatomists and embryologists gave much thought to how disturbances in normal developmental processes might lead to malformations. Lacking the tools of modern microbiology, the early researchers developed some theories which now seem fanciful; perhaps because puerperal infections were then so common, they attributed much embryologic disturbance to infection. Abbott [2] described a number of the early theories in her Atlas and in her other writings. Ferencz [66] has made an interesting tabulation of the etiologic questions posed by Abbott in her Atlas: "Is it true inheritance? Is it altered environment? Is it disease of the early embryo?" and how modern researchers, including herself, have begun to address these questions with modern tools.

Cardiac Defects and Childhood Heart Disease

By the time of publication of Abbott's atlas in 1936, the effect of rheumatic fever on the heart was known. [67] As discussed in chapter 6, the ravages caused by the disease in the Western world were already lessening, and salicylates were in widespread use for therapy of the acute attacks. Other acquired cardiac problems in children, including myocarditis and cardiomyopathy had mostly been the subject of individual case reports. Cardiac medications remained limited to digitalis and mercurial diuretics.

Congenital malformations of the heart were still mainly thought of in terms of pathologic anatomy, [58] but many attempts were made to correlate symptoms, signs, and anatomy. Such correlations were attempted by Ebstein in 1866, and Eisenmenger in 1897. [68,69] Fallot in his series of articles in 1888, [45] opened his essay with the words: "One of those fortunate chances that occasionally are able to provide the clinician with precious opportunities for self-instruction has, in the space of several years, put before our eyes three cases of a rare and curious disease ..." and, alluding to the lack of therapeutic application, "nothing that touches on the solution of a clinical problem, however exceptional ... could be considered as something devoid of interest and without importance." Fallot then analysed the literature and destroyed the prevailing concept that cardiac cyanosis was always due to patency of the foramen ovale. Although it is hard to determine his exact concept of the mechanism causing cyanosis, his essay is a masterpiece of clinical and pathologic description.

When one of us visited Marseilles to participate in the centennial meeting celebrating Fallot's classic paper, it seemed remarkable that Fallot should have been so absorbed by an unusual and untreatable defect. In this vibrant port, in constant communication with both Europe and North Africa, he was in a hot-bed of infectious and social pathology. To our lasting benefit, though he treated many other disorders, his imagination and interest were captured by three exceptional patients. His analysis of their symptoms and intracardiac anatomy, careful review of the literature, and his use of the term "tetralogie" to describe the four anatomic components, made this a wonderful series of papers. [70,71] It is gratifying to note that two of the most eminent cardiac pathologists of our time, Robert Anderson of London and Richard van Praagh of Boston, who are known for having occasional disagreements on nomenclature, nevertheless concur in their praise of Etienne-Louis Arthur Fallot. [72,73]

EARLY DIAGNOSIS OF A SPECIFIC HEART DEFECT

Fallot recorded that in his third patient, a 36 year old cyanotic man, he made a premortem diagnosis:

> *"Blue disease; in our opinion we shall probably find on autopsy the following anatomical lesions: narrowing of the pulmonary artery, intraventricular communication, origin of the aorta displaced to the right, hypertrophy of the right ventricle."*

He remarked without comment that the young man, despite deep cyanosis and clubbing, had been accepted for military service in the Lancers, but invalided out after a few months. Cyanosis had long been recognised as a sign of severe congenital heart disease, probably since the time of Hunter in the mid eighteenth century, but Fallot's report suggests that this concept was not yet widely diffused among physicians screening French Army recruits.

The title of Fallot's paper is in itself intriguing, in implying that "the blue disease" is an interesting contribution only to pathology. New concepts are still evolving from modern studies of the blue disease, using tools unimaginable to Fallot. (Figure 5).

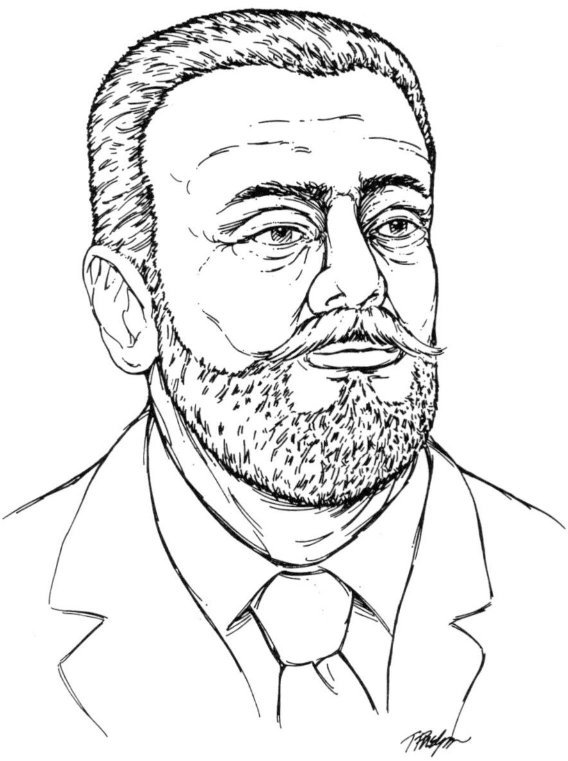

Figure 5—Arthur Fallot (1850–1911) of Marseilles.

The remarkable contribution of Henri Roger has been somewhat diluted by later controversies on ventricular septal defects and the reasons for variability of the physical signs. His demonstration in 1879[51] that the murmur of a ventricular septal defect could be pathognomonic was a major and unassailable conceptual achievement, one which can be better understood now that the defect itself and its characteristic turbulent flow can be visualised with echo-Doppler technology.

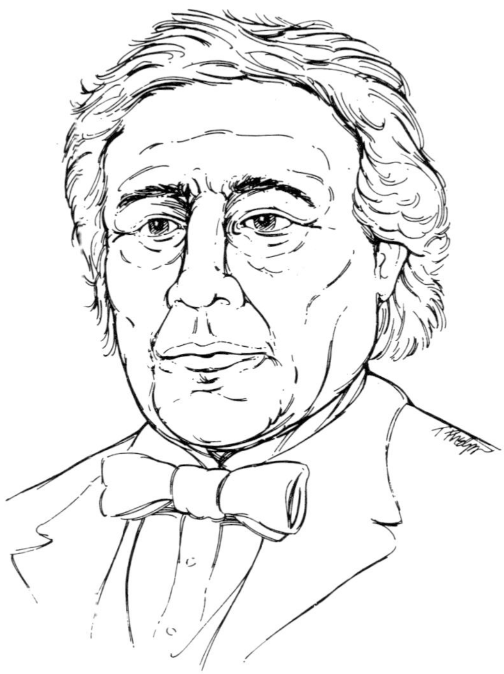

Figure 6 Henri Roger (1809–1891) of Paris.

Gibson of Edinburgh was not the first to recognise the murmur of a patent ductus, which he described in 1900.[53,74,75] However, his paper was remarkable because he expressed his concept of the murmur in physiologic terms:

> *"In consequence of the higher pressure of the blood in the aorta, as compared with the pulmonary artery, there must be a current from the former to the latter, and this stream will be almost, if not quite, continuous ..."*

In many decades of auscultation and teaching, it is unlikely one has heard a more succinct and elegant explanation of this rewarding murmur. He includes an auscultatory diagram in his paper. Although graphic tracings of heart sounds had already been recorded by Einthoven in 1894,[76] Gibson's auscultatory diagram antedated the clinical use of the tool of phonocardiography by at least 30 years.

CLINICOPATHOLOGIC PROFILE

As new tools became available, including chest Xray, [77] fluoroscope, [78] and electrocardiogram, [11,79] they were incorporated into cardiac practice. Thus by 1936 the clinicopathologic profile of tricuspid atresia had been described separately by Brown [80] and by Taussig. [81] Taussig describes in detail how the absence of the normal right ventricular shadow on chest Xray and fluoroscopy in a cyanotic infant, led her to recognise the clinical entity of tricuspid atresia. This was a remarkable combination of astute observation and deductive reasoning; she used the tool of the fluoroscope to study the normal cardiac silhouette, and to deduce the significance of a specific abnormality. Later we will talk of an era of clinicophysiologic correlations. At this time, most of the pioneering correlations were between clinical findings and pathology. A few years later, in 1941, Bedford and associates defined the typical clinical and radiologic findings in atrial septal defect. [82]

Maude Abbott's Atlas [2] owed much of its inspiration to Osler, who urged her to bring a statistical approach to her study of congenital heart defects. Yet a half century later it seems that even more than the statistics of her 1,000 cases, it was her collection from many sources of clinical findings, Xray and electrocardiogram, together with the pathology, which is her most remarkable achievement and enduring monument. This led to the important concept illustrated, though not explicitly stated by her, that a specific clinicopathologic profile existed for each defect.

Abbott (Figure 7) also critically reviewed some theories of cardiac development. Perhaps in retrospect it is easier to see that she was the first person who made the study of childhood heart disease international in scope. Her vigorous

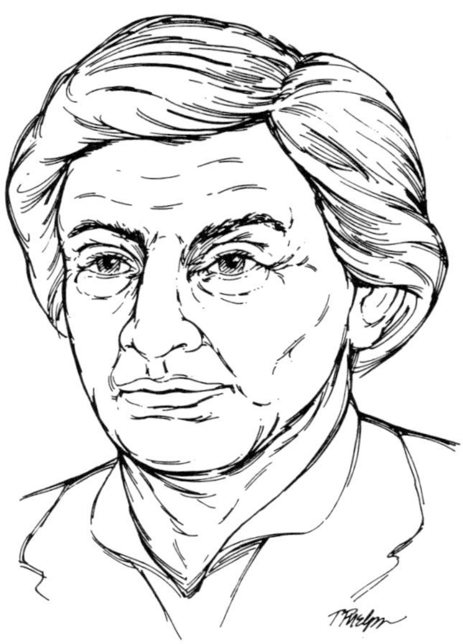

Figure 7—Maude E. Abbott (1869–1940) of Montreal

correspondence with pathologists and clinicians worldwide, her enthusiasm for a subject mostly confined to case reports and pathology museums, brought her affection and esteem, including the honor of being the only woman included in Rivera's amazing mural on medical science in Mexico City. [17]

Preventive Cardiology

Risk factors for adult heart disease were beginning to be thought of, though not yet a focus of medical endeavor. Pickering[83] quotes Frederick Akhbar Mahomed in 1879 on hypertension without renal disease in the young:

> *"... these persons appear to pass through life pretty much as others do, and generally do not suffer from their high blood pressures ... As age advances the enemy gains an accession of strength ... now past forty perhaps fifty years ... he has a cough ... but by his pulse you will know him ... headache, vertigo, a passing paralysis, a more severe apoplectic seizure, and then the final blow."*

Thus the concept that atherosclerosis is progressive with age, and that systemic hypertension begins in youth, with a prolonged silent asymptomatic phase, has a distinguished history, though recognition of the implications for pediatric cardiology have been more recent.

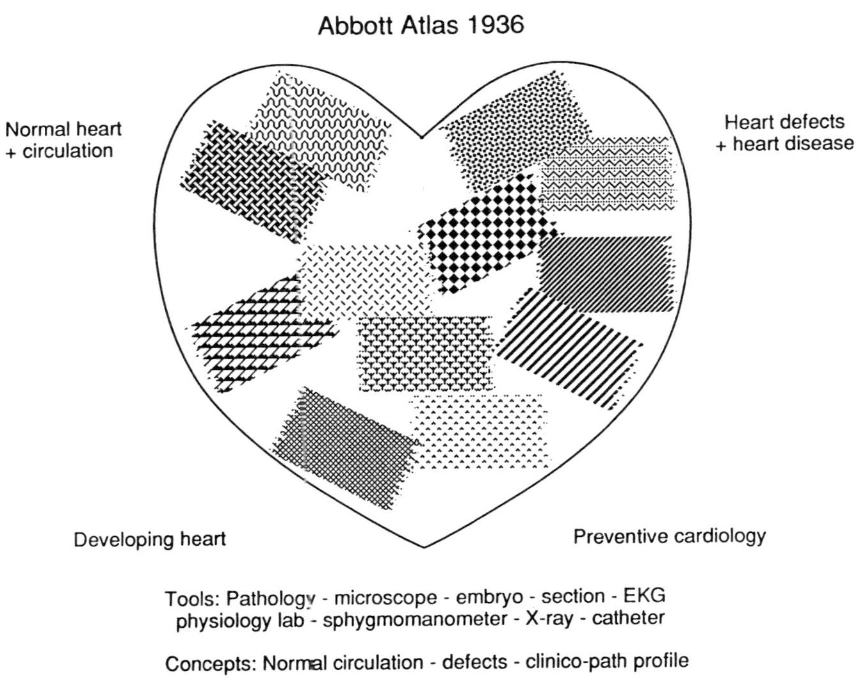

Figure 8—Tools and concepts in 1936 in the 4 domains of pediatric cardiology.

Tools And Concepts in 1936. (Figure 8)

By 1936, the end of the era of pathological anatomy, clinical observations could now be supplemented by chest Xray, fluoroscopy and 6 lead electrocardiogram, though precordial leads were not yet in use.

Physiological studies in laboratories were rapidly extending knowledge of the normal circulation. The measurement of intracardiac pressures was available for animals, but catheter studies of the human heart were in the wings, waiting to emerge as a force in medical history.

Some, indeed most, congenital cardiac malformations had been described pathologically, and for a few, a clinicophysiologic profile was beginning to emerge.

The outline of cardiac development in the embryo had been established. Preventive cardiology was as yet barely a concept, though great advances had been made in the pathology of atherosclerosis, and blood pressure was often measured in adults, though rarely in children.

Thus all four domains of pediatric cardiology had progressed dramatically since the time of Peacock. Some of the tools and concepts available for the study of the hearts of children by 1936 are shown in Figure 8. Pediatric cardiology itself had yet to be born.

The Child with Heart Disease

Pediatrics was now a recognised specialty, and disease in children was now being studied as never before. The true range of childhood heart disease was not yet clear. Although treatment had shown little progress, the world of the child was becoming increasingly recognised as a topic for literature and for new medical approaches.

THE CHILD AND BOOKS

Books had been written for and about children since early in the 15th century. Thinking of the history of pediatric cardiology, one is drawn to consider the amusements, the reading and the world of a child with heart disease before the dawn of therapy.

The late 19th century saw the beginning of a new field of literature, designed for children of different ages, some appealing to childhood love of fantasy, as in the Tales of Beatrix Potter, or Lewis Carroll's Alice in Wonderland. Some dwelt on adventure and exploration, and some, like the stories of Louisa May Alcott, on the interactions of large extended families, with lovable eccentric adults on the periphery, and growing children as their focus and raison d'etre.

Some of the enduring favorites described animals with lives and adventures of their own. This burgeoning of a special branch of reading has many causes, and analysis and literary criticism of such books is now a major research endeavor. It seems certain that the trend was part of a new recognition of the wonder of childhood as a magical part of life, and was inextricably linked with the emerging study of children, their minds, their education, and their health. We are indebted to Catherine Clark, age 11 years, for one of her favorite quotations from a book of this period, Black Beauty. From the time of its first publication in 1877, the book has brought pleasure to healthy children like herself, and to those with heart disease.

> *"My troubles are all over, and I am at home; and often before I am quite awake, I fancy I am still in the orchard at Birtwick with my old friends under the apple trees."*
> —Anna Sewell, Black Beauty 1877

TWO BOYS WITH RHEUMATIC HEART DISEASE

In the late 19th century rheumatic heart disease was rampant among children and young adults. The Harriet Lane Home for Invalid Children, later to be the site of Helen Taussig's cardiac clinic, was founded in 1912. The funds for the building, a separate structure on the grounds of the Johns Hopkins Hospital, were donated by Harriet Lane Johnston, niece of President Buchanan, and her husband, to commemorate their two sons who had died of rheumatic fever in their early teens. Little appears to have been written of these children, who illustrate that rheumatic fever was at one time a killer disease in the Western world, one not confined to the poor.

The Harriet Lane Home was far from being the first children's hospital, being preceded by those in Florence, London and many other centers around the world. It is, however, remarkable that these two tragic young deaths inspired the building of a structure where so much cardiac history would later be made. Harriet Lane Johnston, who died many years after her husband, also left money in her will for the St Albans choir school at Washington National Cathedral, to commemorate that her sons, during their brief lives, had been choristers at St Pauls Church in Baltimore. A window in St Pauls Church is dedicated to them, with the words:

To the glory of God and in blessed memory of
James Buchanan Johnston
Whom God took unto Himself Annunciation Day 1881 in the 15th year of his age

and of Henry Elliot Johnston
whom God also took unto himself Oct 30th 1882 in the 13th year of his age

A memorial from their loving parents.
We asked life of them and Thou gavest them a long life even for ever and ever.

Many parents of many faiths and lands have lost children to heart disease since these words were written. The Johnstons were able to commemorate their children in perpetuity. One hopes they would have been happy to know that a century later, rheumatic fever is a disappearing disease, at least in the Western world.

A FAMOUS PEDIATRICIAN'S VIEW OF A CONGENITAL HEART DEFECT

For the child born with a congenital heart defect, as we have tried to show, many conceptual advances had already been made, but it is uncertain if these advances were widely known, or often affected the interaction of physician and child.

During the last 70 years of the pretherapeutic era, the years from Peacock to Abbott, the concept of a clinical profile had been growing steadily. Yet the atmosphere of therapeutic nihilism which prevailed outside centers of specialised interest is perhaps conveyed most vividly by the physician writer William Carlos Williams in 1933. While making a home visit to the subject of his story "The girl with a pimply face," he was asked to examine her sister, a sick little infant who had just been discharged from a New Jersey hospital where she had acquired gastroenteritis and a severe diaper rash, but apparently no diagnosis or treatment.

> *"There it lay, just skin and bones with a round fleshless head at the top and the usual pot belly you find in such cases ... It had no temperature. There was no rash. The mouth was in reasonably good shape. Eyes, ears negative. The moment I put my stethoscope to the little boney chest, however, the whole thing became clear. The infant had a severe congenital heart defect, a roar when you listened over the heart that meant, to put it crudely, that she was no good, never would be."*

> William Carlos Williams: *The Doctor Stories.* Copyright 1938 by William Carlos Williams. Reprinted by permission of New Directions Publishing Corp.

Reading the story 60 years after it was written, one remains glad that at a later visit the infant was reported "better," indeed doing well. Perhaps, using the retrospectoscope, one can surmise she had a membranous ventricular septal defect which underwent spontaneous decrease in size. She was born six years before Gross successfully ligated a patent ductus, about 20 years before the introduction of banding of the pulmonary artery, almost 40 years before successful surgical closure of ventricular septal defects in infancy, and almost 30 years before John Keith's group in Toronto brought back to life the concept that some such defects may close spontaneously. Perhaps she is still living happily in Rutherford New Jersey, and has children and even grandchildren of her own.

The story illustrates that although knowledge had advanced dramatically, there was still no effective therapy. The approach to diagnosis of congenital heart defects by a good primary care physician in 1933 had not advanced greatly since the time when Farre, in 1814, lamented the conceptual poverty of a simple diagnosis of "heart disease."

ADDITIONAL REFERENCES AND NOTES

47. Fye WB. Growth of American Physiology 1850-1900. In: Physiology in the American context, 1850-1940 American Physiological Society 1987: 47-65.

48. Pohlman AG. The course of the blood through the heart of the fetal mammal, with a note on the reptilian and amphibian circulations. Anatomical Record 1909;3:75-109.

49. Melka J. Beitrag zur Kenntnis der Morphologie und Obliteration des Ductus arteriosus Botalli. Anat Anzeiger 1926;61:348-360.

50. Fick A. Ueber die Messung des Blutquantums in den Herzventrikeln. Phys-Med Geselle Wurzburg Sitzungber. 1870:16.

51. Roger H. Recherches cliniques sur la communication congenitale des deux coeurs, par inocclusion de septum interventriculaire. Bull de l'Acad Medecin 1879;8:1077-1085.

52. Keith A, Flack M. The form and nature of the muscular connections between the primary divisions of the vertebrate heart. J Anat Physiol 1907:41:172-189.

53. Gibson GA. Persistence of the arterial duct and its diagnosis. Edinburgh Med J 1900;8:1-3.

54. Starling EH. The Linacre Lecture on the Law of the Heart given at Cambridge, 1915. London, Longmans Green, 1918.

55. Chaveau A, Marey EJ. Determination graphique des rapports du choc du coeur avec les mouvements des oreillettes et des ventricles: experience faite a l'aide a un appareil enregistreur (sphygmographe) C.R. Hebd Acad Sci 1861;53:662.

55a. Snellen HA. EJ Marey and cardiology. Rotterdam, Kooyker, 1980.

56. Forssmann W. Die Sonderung des rechter Herzens. Klinische Wochenschrift 1929;8:2085-2087.

57. His W. Das Herz. In: Anatomie menschlicher Embryonen. Theil 3: Zur Geschichte der Organe. Leipzig, Vogel, 1885.

58. Rokitansky CF von. Die Defekte der Scheidewande des Herzens. Pathologisch-Anatomische. Vienna, Wilhelm Braumuller, 1875.

59. Grant RT. The development of the cardiac coronary vessels in the rabbit. Heart 1926;13:261-271.

60. Davis CL. Development of the human heart from its first appearance to the stage found in embryos of twenty paired somites. Carnegie Contributions to Embryology 1927:19-107-247-293.

61. Van Mierop LHS. Morphological development of the heart. In Handbook of Physiology, Section 2, Volume I, Berne RM editor. American Physiological Society, Bethesda. 1979:1-28.

62. Mall FP. On stages in the development of human embryos from 2 to 25 mm long. Anatomische Anzeiger 1914;46:78-84.

63. Streeter GL. Developmental Horizons in Human Embryos. Age Groups XI to XXIII. In Contributions to Embryology, reprint #2. Heuser CH, Corner GW, editors. Washington, Carnegie Institute of Washington, 1951.

64. O'Rahilly R, Muller F. Developmental Stages in Human Embryos: Including a Revision of Streeter's "Horizons" and a Survey of the Carnegie Collection. In: Carnegie Institute of Washington Publication #637,1987.

65. Horder TJ. The emergence of experimental embryology in Germany. In: A History of Embryology. Horder TJ, Witkowski JA, Wylie CC editors. Cambridge, Cambridge University Press 1986:179-182.

66. Ferencz C. Origin of congenital heart disease: Reflections on Maude Abbott's work. Canadian J Cardiol 1989;5:4-9.

67. Cheadle WB. The Various Manifestations of the Rheumatic State as Exemplified in Childhood and Early Life. London, Smith Elder, 1889.

68. Ebstein W. Uber einem sehr seltener Fall von Insufficienz der Valvula Tricuspidalis, bedingt durch ein angeborene hochgradige Missbildung derselben. Arch Anat Physiol Wissenshaftl 1866;33:238-254.

69. Eisenmenger V. Die angeborenen Defecte der Kammerscheidewand des Herzens. Zeitscrift Klinische Medizin. 1897;32 (suppl):1-28.

70. Gerard R. Un centenaire:la tetralogie de Fallot 1888-1988. Arch Mal Coeur Vaiss 1988;81:1313-1315.

71. Allwork SP. Tetralogy of Fallot: the centenary of the name. A new translation of the first of Fallot's papers. Eur J Cardiothoracic Surg 1988;2:386-392.

72. Anderson RH, Tynan M. Tetralogy of Fallot-a centennial review. [Review] Int J Cardiol 1988;21: 219-232.

73. Van Praagh R. Etienne-Louis Arthur Fallot and his tetralogy: a new translation of Fallot's summary and a modern reassessment of this anomaly. Eur J Cardiothoracic Surg 1989;3:381-386.

74. Duroziez P. Memoire sur la persistance du canal arteriel sans autre communication anormale. Memoires de la Societe de Biologie: Comptes Rendus. 1862;4:279-292.

75. Cassels DE. The patent ductus arteriosus: I. Historical aspects of clinical recognition of patency. In The Ductus Arteriosus. Cassels DE, editor. Springfield, Charles C Thomas, 1973: 104-142.

76. Caceres CA, Perry LW. Principles of Phonocardiography. In: The innocent murmur: A problem in clinical practice. Boston, Little Brown, 1967: 45-61.

77. Rontgen WC. On a new kind of rays. Nature 1896;53:274-276.

78. Williams FH. A method for more fully determining the outline of the heart by means of a fluorescope (sic), together with other uses of this instrument in medicine. Boston Med Surg J 1896; 135: 335-337.

79. Einthoven W. Le telecardiogramme. Arch Inst Physiol 1906;4:132-164.

80. Brown JW. Congenital tricuspid atresia. Arch Dis Child 1936;11:275-278.

81. Taussig HB. Clinical and pathologic findings in congenital malformations of the heart due to defective development of the right ventricle associated with tricuspid atresia or hypoplasia. Bull Johns Hopkins Hosp 1936;59:435-444.

82. Bedford DE, Papp C, Parkinson J. Atrial septal defect. Brit Heart J 1941;3:37-68.

83. Pickering G. Systemic arterial hypertension. In: Circulation of the Blood: Men and Ideas. Fishman AP, Richards DW, editors. New York, Oxford Univ. Press, 1964:501.

CHAPTER 4

The Dawn of Therapy 1936-1955

- Closed heart surgery (PDA/Blalock Taussig shunt/coarctation)
- Role of fluoroscopy
- Tools of cardiac catheterisation, angiocardiography
- Interaction of clinicophysiologic concepts and surgery

Introduction

The age of therapy dawned only two years after the publication of Abbott's Atlas. Dr William Gross, at that time a surgical Resident at the Childrens Hospital in Boston, ligated a patent ductus arteriosus on August 26 1938 [84]. The concept of clinicophysiologic correlation had already been introduced, but the advent of surgery gave diagnosis an impetus and immediacy which had been lacking before. Repair of aortic coarctation and the development of the Blalock Taussig shunt followed soon afterwards, and by the end of the 1940s closed heart surgery was available for many defects. The period from 1936 to 1955 was the dawn of therapy, the beginning of a completely new way of viewing congenital heart defects as capable of diagnosis, understanding, and treatment.

By 1938, the year Gross began closed heart surgery, opening of the chest was no longer prohibitively risky. Pneumonectomies had already been performed, and there had been occasional successes with the Trendeleburg operation for pulmonary embolectomy [12,13]. Anesthesia was still primitive by today's standards, but was already in use throughout the Western world. October 11 1846 was celebrated as "Ether Day," and schools of anesthesia had been established. Brieger has given a scholarly account of some of these advances, which formed an essential background to the arrival of the modern era of therapy [85].

Prior to the period of intense activity which now began, interest in cardiac surgery had been limited by technical considerations, by long standing admonitions against intruding on the heart, and by limited understanding of therapeutic goals.

During the almost 20 years between the first ligation of a patent ductus in 1938 and the advent of cardiopulmonary bypass in 1955, surgeons and anesthetists refined their skills, and the new discipline of pediatric cardiology was born. New diagnostic and therapeutic tools came into use, and the establishment of cardiac catheterisation laboratories ushered in an era of clinicophysiologic correlations. Diagnosis came to include more than simple anatomic definition of a cardiac defect, but began to involve concepts of the range of hemodynamic severity. Clinicophysiologic profiles were established for most defects. The tools of Xray, electrocardiogram, and later, cardiac catheterisation, helped to define the spectrum of severity of a number of cardiac problems.

THE INTERACTION OF SURGERY AND CLINICOPHYSIOLOGIC CORRELATION

The impetus for this new era came from successful surgery, with duct ligation, coarctation repair, and the Blalock Taussig shunt following rapidly after one another. The ability to treat previously untouchable lesions spurred intense interest in accurate diagnosis, and in methods of correlating physiology with clinical findings. For example, now that a ductus could be ligated, it became of more than academic interest to ask "Is there always a continuous murmur with a patent ductus? What may modify the murmur? What other defect might cause a continuous murmur?" In 1938 none of these questions could be answered, and indeed had never been asked. Thus surgery stimulated a widespread search for clinicophysiologic correlations, and as physiologic understanding grew, further surgery was conceptualised and undertaken. This mutual stimulation of physiologic, clinical and surgical concepts continued for many decades.

Direct observation of a defect at surgery was very different from the previous attempts to correlate clinical findings with anatomy after the heart was no longer beating. The surgeon could feel the continuous thrill over the patent ductus, and observe its disappearance with duct ligation. A sense of immediacy had entered cardiology.

THE AGE OF THERAPY

The first era in the therapeutic age, the clinicophysiologic-surgical era from 1940-1975, will occupy numerous future historians, and only a few highlights will be mentioned here. Many of the major contributions have been collected and analysed [4,7,9,12,13,86,87]. William Glenn, himself one of the important surgical pioneers, has a history of cardiac surgery on permanent exhibit in the medical library at Yale-New Haven [88].

The second era of infant diagnosis and treatment from 1975-1990 is still in progress, and further management advances will occur. In the third, the current developmental era starting in the 1990's, the major focus lies with increased understanding of the heart at the molecular level, and on more sophisticated analyses of outcome and prognosis.

In this chapter we will analyse some of the changes in pediatric cardiology between 1939 and 1955. During the almost two decades separating the first duct ligation from the beginning of open heart surgery in 1955, many children were successfully treated, and the study of the hearts of children spread around the world.

The Normal Cardiovascular System

By the beginning of the age of therapy the tools of chest Xray and fluoroscopy had established standards of normal heart size in adults and children. Methods of recognising specific chamber enlargement were well defined. The electrocardiogram was in use, and some differences between childhood and adult electrocardiographic patterns were beginning to be recognised.

In animal laboratories intensive physiologic study of the heart and circulation, using increasingly sophisticated tools, were undertaken in the decades between the 1930s and 1950s.

The tool of cardiac catheterisation, developed for use in animals in the nineteenth century, was later used experimentally on himself by Forssman [56]. The procedure began to be used in the study of childhood heart disease in the mid 1940s [42,89-91]. Gradually the normal cardiac output at various ages was documented.

In 1939 Barclay and colleagues published the first accounts of the fetal circulation in animals, using both catheterisation and angiocardiographic techniques [92]. Their work opened the whole new research field of fetal physiology.

Jesse Edwards, then at the Mayo Clinic, was among the first to show changes in the pulmonary vascular bed of neonates [93]. This work, published in 1951, began the evolution of new concepts of the interrelationship of neonatal physiology with pulmonary arteriolar changes. This interrelationship was studied in the 1950's by James and Rowe [94] after the introduction of cardiac catheterisation in infants. Their pioneering research was the stimulus to many subsequent investigations of neonatal cardiopulmonary physiology.

The Developing Heart

Cardiac embryology was now being studied in laboratories all over the world, though most of the researchers continued to come from the disciplines of anatomy and biology. Prior to the mid 1950s there were few formal affiliations between clinicians working with childhood heart disease and those studying embryology. Snellen's group in Leiden was one of the few where active interchange occured [14]. One of us (CAN) was fortunate to work at the Carnegie Institute of Embryology for a year while the Streeter collection of serially sectioned hearts was still housed in Baltimore. The scholarly and talented group assembled there by the then Director, Dr George Corner, never expressed surprise that a pediatric cardiologist of that day might temporarily pose as an embryologist. Perhaps the happiness and memories of that year now make it possible, to quote Rashkind, to have the audacity to be a "pediatric cardiologist posing as a historian!" [24,95].

In later years, of course, starting in the 1970's, a number of ambitious studies in embryology and molecular biology were undertaken by pediatric cardiologists, who became recognised as distinguished investigators in early growth of the heart; some of these projects are discussed in later chapters.

Cardiac Defects and Childhood Heart Disease

Heart problems in infants and children emerged from the chrysalis phase of quiet study and analytic thought on to center stage in medical history. The change came with dramatic suddenness. Although there had been a steady increase in knowledge of many aspects of pediatric cardiology, including understanding of clinicophysiologic concepts, the sudden change came from new therapy, in the dawn of cardiac surgery.

THE DAWN OF CARDIAC SURGERY

The dawn of heart surgery had been slow in coming [12,13,88]. Some surgeons, including Harvey Cushing, had expressed optimism in the late nineteenth century that surgery on heart valves would one day be possible. But most surgical teaching stressed the hazards of approaching the heart. The pericardium had been successfully sutured a few times in the late 19th century, but Bilroth, a towering surgical figure in Europe, is quoted to have said "A surgeon who tries to suture a heart wound deserves to lose the esteem of his colleagues." [13]. Stephen Paget in 1896 wrote a textbook on Surgery of the Chest [96], an achievement that should, one would think, have brought him praise for being a pioneer. It is his ill fortune, and a warning to all of us who attempt to write books, that the only statement from the book which is ever quoted is his prediction:

> *"Surgery of the heart has probably reached the limits set by nature to all surgery: no new method and no new discovery can overcome the natural difficulties that attend a wound of the heart. It is true that heart suture has been vaguely proposed as a possible procedure, and that it has been done in animals, but I cannot find that it has ever been attempted in practice." [96]*

Only a few months after Paget's pessimistic statement was published, in September 1896, Ludwig Rehn of Frankfurt Germany succesfully sutured a heart wound of the right ventricle [97]. The patient was a 22 year old man who had been stabbed with a knife "in the fourth interspace, three fingersbreadths to the left of the sternal margin." The wound was 1.4 cm long, and Rehn describes the blood distending the pericardium, and how bleeding was greater in systole than diastole. "The wound was closed with three silk sutures placed during several diastolic phases. The pulse was immediately improved." Iodoform gauze drains were placed in the pleural and pericardial spaces. The young man recovered and was able to return to work.

Since Rehn's low key description of this remarkable event, a number of other surgeons had ventured into the treacherous area of repair of cardiac wounds and relief of cardiac tamponade. A few had attempted mitral valvotomy, and many advances in thoracic surgery were made treating the wounded in Europe in the latter part of World War II [12,13,88].

Modern cardiac surgery began with the ligation of a patent arterial duct in a seven year old girl [84]. Pediatric anesthesia and surgery were still very new, and although thoracotomy, primarily used for pulmonary tuberculosis, had a longer history, the heroic nature of the procedure is impressive. The brief and classic paper by Gross and Hubbard documents a 40mm mercury rise in diastolic blood pressure postoperatively; the statement that the child had been seen in several different hospitals between three and seven years of age, with the same diagnosis in all, "congenital malformation of the heart with a patent ductus arteriosus," suggests that the clinical profile of a large patent ductus was now already a part of general pediatric knowledge.

THE BLALOCK TAUSSIG ANASTOMOSIS

In the same year of 1939, the year of publication of Gross and Hubbard's paper [84], Alfred Blalock had already performed a subclavian-pulmonary artery anastomosis in the dog in an effort to produce pulmonary hypertension [98,99]. This work, performed at Vanderbilt, preceded Blalock's move to Johns Hopkins. Alfred Blalock came to Johns Hopkins as Professor of Surgery in 1941, accompanied by his research laboratory assistant Vivien Thomas.

By 1941 Helen Taussig already had a large pediatric cardiac clinic, and used the fluoroscope as a major tool of diagnosis: in the preface to the second edition of her textbook [18] she pays tribute to Blalock "who took my work beyond the realm of academic interest and made it of vital importance" and to "Dr Edwards A. Park to whom I am indebted for my life's work ... He put me in charge of the cardiac clinic and gave me the tools with which to work ... In 1930 he had a fluoroscope installed in the Harriet Lane Home with instructions to USE IT."

The tool of the fluoroscope was essential to Helen Taussig's concept that in most cyanotic children, particularly those with tetralogy of Fallot, the pulmonary vascularity was reduced and more flow to the lungs was needed [42]. Although pulmonary stenosis was a recognised anatomic component of tetralogy, the fluoroscope made the physiologic impact much more vivid. She was thus able to separate out a group of cyanotic children with decreased pulmonary vascular markings who might be helped.

The fluoroscope alone would of course have been worthless without the conceptual genius which led to the idea of bypassing the right ventricular outflow obstruction. Taussig's concept of the benefit of an "artificial ductus" arose from observing that cyanosis increased and cyanotic spells began some weeks after birth, changes she attributed to closure of the ductus.

Vivien Thomas, the technically brilliant research associate who had accompanied Dr. Blalock to Baltimore, wrote a fascinating account of his experiences both in the laboratory, and in the city where desegregation was still evolving [99]. He describes a meeting with Taussig and Blalock one morning in 1943 where Taussig "expressed her belief that, by surgical means, it should be possible to do something

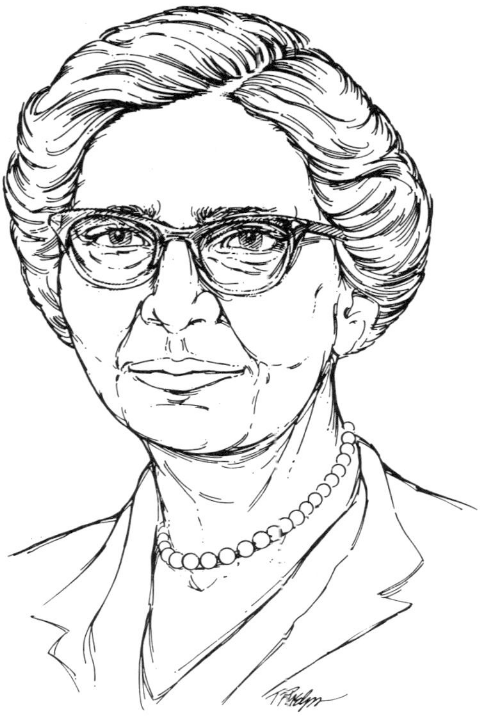

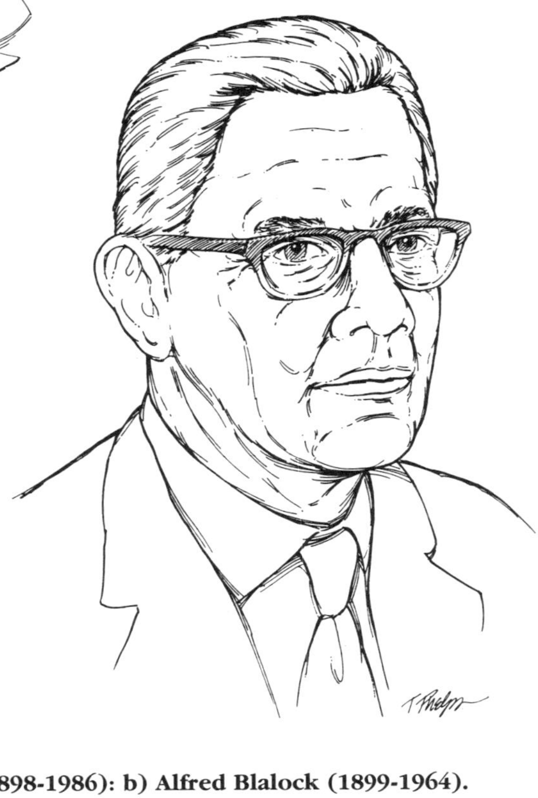

Figure 9—a) Helen Brooke Taussig (1898-1986): b) Alfred Blalock (1899-1964).

to get more blood to the lungs." The concepts and tools available to the trio at that meeting (Figure 9) led to one of the most remarkable events in the history of pediatric cardiology, the first successful treatment of cyanotic heart disease [100].

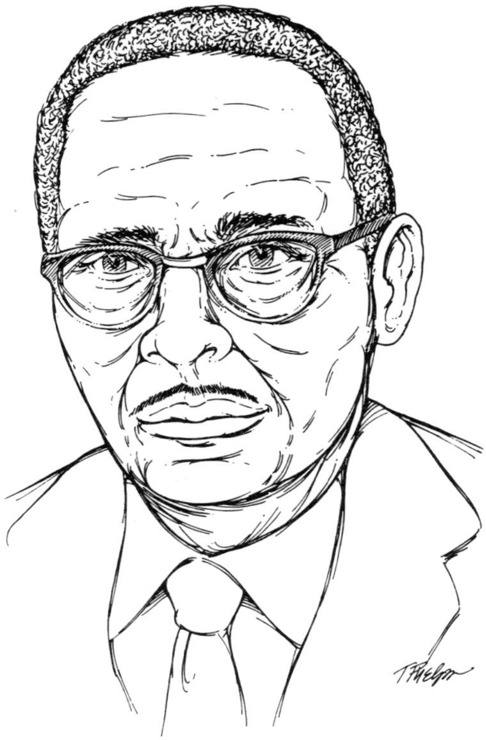

Figure 9—c) Vivien Thomas (1910-1989).

In their first paper Blalock and Taussig describe with considerable clinical detail the first three patients to undergo this new operation. The figure below, which is redrawn from the original illustration, shows not only the anastomosis, but an inset sketch of a child and a chest incision.

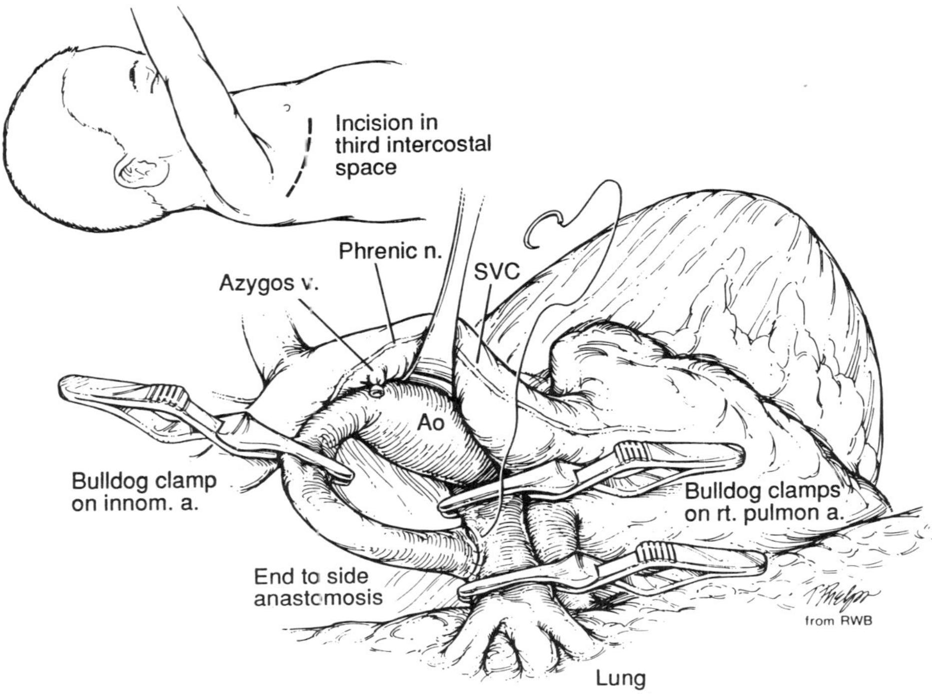

Figure 10—Blalock Taussig anastomosis. Redrawn from original illustration JAMA 1945 [100]: courtesy Medical Archives Johns Hopkins Medical Institutions.

Ruth Whittemore, later of New Haven, was Helen Taussig's major assistant in the early years after the first shunt procedure. She had obtained her M.D. degree at Johns Hopkins in 1942, and in November 1944, as a pediatric resident, was entrusted with the postoperative care of the first child to undergo the new operation. She gave a brief description of the experience in a recent interview for the Hopkins Advocate [101], quoted below:

> *"It was a girl, Eileen Saxon," Dr Whittemore relates today, as fifty years slip away. "She came out of surgery with numerous postoperative complications. I had to stick needles into both sides of her chest to draw off air that was compressing her lungs." For two days Whittemore was in constant attendance, sleeping on a stretcher near the baby. "We didn't have a way to monitor the pressure on her lungs, so I rigged up a way to monitor it without having to stick her repeatedly. It was definitely a Rube Goldberg affair, but the baby came through it.*
>
> *As for me, I fell into pediatric cardiology and couldn't get out."*

After "falling into" pediatric cardiology, Ruth Whittemore was Helen Taussig's senior Fellow and first assistant before leaving in 1947 to become the first Director of pediatric cardiology at the Yale-New Haven Medical Center. In the same interview [101] she describes how cyanotic and limited were many of the 400 children waiting to see her when she arrived at Yale. She started pediatric cardiac catheterisation there, and set up a state-wide program for children with rheumatic and congenital heart disease. With her surgical colleagues, Harris B. Shumaker Jr, and later William W. Glenn, she made many contributions to the field, particularly in follow up of the "second generation," the children of parents born to those with heart defects [102].

At the time Ruth Whittemore sat by the bedside of Eileen Saxon, everything was new. Since thoracotomies had so rarely been performed in childhood, pediatric anesthesia and postoperative care were only beginning. A number of accounts have been written of those early years, and many more will be written in future. We asked Dr Henry Bahnson, who has already published a retrospection on some of his experiences [103], to give us some personal memories from a perspective of almost 50 years later. Henry Bahnson, a long time friend and former colleague, worked at Johns Hopkins with Dr Blalock for many years before becoming Chairman and Chief of Cardiovascular Surgery at the University of Pittsburgh. He has allowed us to quote some of his memories of those years, years when the long, productive, and sometimes testy partnership of cardiac surgery and pediatric cardiology was being born.

Memories: beginning of an era. Henry T. Bahnson M.D.

"On November 30, 1944, at the Johns Hopkins Hospital, I rotated as an unsuspecting intern to the surgical service that included, among other duties, care of children undergoing an operation. Fresh from an accelerated three years in medical school, and planning after the war to return to North Carolina to practice general surgery, I was unaware that on the previous day the opening wedge had been made that would open the avenue to my future work and lead to many new fields of medical and surgical endeavor. On that day Alfred Blalock had anastomosed the left subclavian artery of Eileen Saxon to her pulmonary artery in order to treat her tetralogy of Fallot. She was not doing famously, and Dr Blalock, Helen Taussig, Bill Longmire (the chief surgical resident) and Ruth Whittemore (pediatric Fellow) were frequently at the bedside and oxygen tent. The latter was about the only special treatment available postoperatively. It was remarkable that the fifteen month old, frail, cyanotic, 4 Kg child was still alive. The operation had been done with open drop ether given by Merle Harmel M.D., and the end-to-side anastomosis was done with small, straight, milliner's needles threaded with "china beaded silk." Pneumo- and hemo-thorax were treated with needle thoracentesis. (No chest tube was placed). She survived remarkably, as did two other young patients and all were improved before the first report in the JAMA of May 1945. Although at that time constrictive pericarditis, lacerations, and tamponade of the heart were being treated—Dr Blalock had made major contributions to their understanding—and Robert Gross had interrupted a patent ductus in a number of patients, this was a pivotal opening event of the surgery for cardiac abnormalities and for the later development of many related specialties.

... Helen Taussig, who had a special and consuming interest in pediatric cardiology, recognised the significance of a patent ductus arteriosus in ameliorating the condition of a patient with the tetralogy of Fallot and had earlier asked Robert Gross of Boston Children's Hospital if he could create rather than interrupt a ductus. Gross had apparently

unproductively discussed the matter with his colleagues because I recall a discussion of it by Dr Sidney Farber at Children's with my Harvard Medical School Pathology section in 1942 or 1943.

Soon after Blalock arrived as Chairman of Surgery at Hopkins, Dr Edwards A. Park, Chairman of Pediatrics, asked Blalock if he could do anything about coarctation of the aorta. Characteristically, Dr Blalock went to the laboratory and devised a technique of swinging the left subclavian artery, divided at its distal end, around the isthmus (which is the usual site of coarctation) and anastomosing it to the aorta distally. In a short time Blalock returned with a report of finished experimental work on dogs and a completed manuscript on which Park was listed as a coauthor. Dr Park unsuccessfully objected to being made a coauthor when he had merely made a suggestion, but he also recognised and told Blalock that this was the answer to Taussig's quest.

Again characteristically, Blalock turned to the laboratory and attempted to produce and correct cyanotic animals. He was only partially successful in producing cyanosis and diminished pulmonary blood flow, but much in the first publication with Taussig has to do with the physiology of cyanosis and diminished pulmonary blood flow ..."

Bahnson goes on to describe Blalock's generosity towards his colleagues and especially his residents. Although Blalock did not seek publicity, there was an influx of patients, obviously ill, cyanotic, and limited, who were going to Hopkins and returning home pink, active and healthy. There was much publicity and Bahnson especially recalled a prominent article in the widely read *Saturday Evening Post.* "Such publicity was foreign to custom, practice and even ethics of the time." When Blalock presented his experiences with 110 patients at the American Surgical Association, he was criticised in some opening remarks by the Association president for the publicity, and was with difficulty persuaded not to resign. "His presentation later in the meeting was received with unprecedently enthusiastic applause." Bahnson continues:

"As it turns out that November day in 1944 ws pivotal for me also. When I returned from the Pacific eighteen months later, approximately 200 of the operations had been done. The chief Resident had helped Dr Blalock or Bill Longmire on almost all of these and was finding it exceedingly difficult to complete his own work in addition to the load of blue babies. They looked for someone who could be "dedicated" to help Dr Blalock, and I was the most easily expendable person. Assigned exclusively to work with the hearts, I helped on the next 200 or so patients. I worked out a small laboratory experiment that involved the subclavian-pulmonary anastomosis and soon learned to do the procedure on dogs alone. In time, Dr Blalock helped me to do a number of the operations on patients before I had done more than very few other operations such as hernias and appendectomies which were the usual teaching procedures. When Dr and Mary Blalock went to Europe, he as a visiting professor at Guy's Hospital in London, I was asked to go as an assistant and was accompanied by my wife Louise. It was like riding on the back of Dr Blalock's cresting wave. At the end of the trip, after a number of successful operations in London and Paris, Dr Blalock left me at the hospital to do a patent ductus, the first to be operated on in Paris, while he toured the Tuileries gardens. He said he was tired of working, but he was characteristically giving me the opportunity. I was then three years out of medical school.

Diagnosis of congenital heart disease at that time depended upon history, physical examination, electrocardiography, principally fluoroscopic radiography and roentgenography. Taussig was adept at all of these in spite of her deafness and use of electrical amplification (for her stethoscope). Two other avenues of clinical investigation and research began then and developed strikingly since. Blalock brought Richard Bing to the department of surgery to set up a clinical research laboratory. Bing soon saw a fertile field and pioneered in development of a catheterisation lab. During their first procedure on a 4 or 5 year old boy, he and Vivien Thomas were alarmed when the catheter left the cardiac shadow as seen on the fluoroscope and went into the lung field. They thought they had perforated the heart, but as they soon realised the catheter had simply traversed an atrial septal defect into a pulmonary vein. Similarly for some time almost every study gave previously unknown information, and Bing and his colleagues charted the foundation in congenital heart disease of what has become invasive cardiology.

Angiocardiography came later and had a day in the sun before being combined with catheterisation and central injection of contrast material. Mark Ravitch in 'Alfred Blalock 1889-1964' [86] describes this better than I can: 'In spite of his many, often daring, contributions to surgical concepts and practice, Blalock's attitude towards new departures in medicine was one of thoughtful conservatism. When he and E. D. Churchill were to address the New York Academy of Medicine, he took Hanlon and Bahnson with him to New York to see Sussman's angiocardiographic apparatus. He developed no enthusiasm for the process. However, Hanlon and Bahnson took it on as their problem to work on, nights and weekends, in the old wood floored surgical building erected for Halsted in 1904, in which the department of radiology was then - miserably - housed. Bahnson, on a Christmas visit to his home in Winston Salem, North Carolina, himself had made - with angle irons and a track on which ten cassettes slid beneath a table propelled by a rope and pulley activated by great counterweight and controlled by a solenoid valve to allow the exposed cassette to drop off into a box as the next cassette was pulled into place-the first rapid cassette changer at the Johns Hopkins Hospital.

At times the solenoid release would jam in the open position, permitting the cassettes to thunder uninterruptedly into the box on the floor, assaulting the ears and nerves of patients and surgeons alike; at other times it would fail to open, so that Bahnson regularly crouched half under the table, one hand grasping the plunger of the solenoid as he leaned hopefully out of the direct Xray beam'" [86].

Bahnson concludes: *"From these early beginnings what progress, challenges, and joys the last half century has brought!"*

Tools and Concepts We have already discussed briefly Helen Taussig's extraordinary concept that cyanosis and symptoms would be relieved by increasing blood flow to the lungs. Another concept seldom referred to in discussing the pioneer years is the crucial one of accurate diagnosis. How did Helen Taussig <u>know</u> that Eileen Saxon had tetralogy of Fallot?

The first cardiac catheterisation was done at Johns Hopkins in 1946, two years after ES had surgery: angiocardiography started in a separate laboratory in the same year, 1946. The first pediatric echocardiogram was performed in 1973, long after Helen Taussig's retirement, and decades after over 1,000 Blalock Taussig anastomoses had been performed at Johns Hopkins and many thousands more world wide.

The concept that tetralogy can be diagnosed prior to Doppler echocardiography may bring a look of bored incredulity or open scepticism to the face of the modern medical student or pediatric resident. There is, indeed, no present urgent need or outstanding merit in such a feat, although a good clinician will always wish to use the tool of echocardiography to confirm a diagnosis rather than to initiate one. From a historical viewpoint however, the question, "how did she know?," is of interest.

Fallot himself drew attention to the preponderance of his tetralogy among cyanotic patients surviving beyond infancy. Abbott re-emphasised this, maintaining that tetralogy accounted for at least 70% of the cyanotic group. The clinical profile included, in addition to cyanosis, a cardiac systolic murmur and thrill along the left sternal border, a boot shaped heart with reduced pulmonary vascular markings on chest Xray and fluoroscopy, and right axis deviation on the electrocardiogram. Any divergence from this pattern, whether increased pulmonary vascular markings or left axis deviation, was overwhelmingly against the diagnosis of tetralogy, which had a rather consistent clinicophysiologic profile, particularly in the severely affected children seeking help in the early years.

Helen Taussig was not only familiar with the clinical picture, she had been following infants and children with heart defects in her clinic for twelve years before the first shunt procedure. To her, tetralogy was not a series of old historic articles, but a reality in children she already knew and loved.

Although cyanotic spells had been described by many, Taussig seems to have been the first to add squatting on exertion as being characteristic. (One of us later referred to it as the "coffee shop sign," since if one came into Johns Hopkins past the hospital coffee shop early in the morning, a young child might be seen squatting on a chair to eat breakfast. Not pathognomonic, but highly suggestive. Now, of course, this sign does not occur in the Western world, since cardiac repair in infancy is the rule).

A right aortic arch was already described as being much more common in tetralogy than in other defects, and Taussig used to describe a journey she made to visit Maude Abbott to learn how to diagnose a right aortic arch on barium swallow. Helen Taussig was able to make the correct diagnosis, and ultimately to teach others how to do so, by a combination of experience, skilled use of the building blocks of the tools she had, a knowledge of probabilities, and in her case, an unrivalled clinical genius. She was the unequalled seamstress of the patchwork quilt which is the history of pediatric cardiology.

What Did the Blalock Taussig Shunt Accomplish? Now that shunts are rarely performed, and then mainly as temporising palliative procedures in infants who do not have typical tetralogy (i.e. either have tetralogy with pulmonary atresia or some very complex defect), it is difficult to visualise the excitement the operation caused.

A letter from 12 year old Jean-Pierre Cablan, kept framed by Helen Taussig on her mantelpiece and reproduced in her book [18], expresses some of the drama of those early days. After many long centuries cyanosis could be reversed, a child, in Taussig's phrase, was changed from "blue to pink." Jean-Pierre wrote "Je suis maintenant un tout autre petit garcon ... je vais pouvoir aller jouer avec mes petits camarades." The letter expressed for her, her guests and for posterity, not only the joy of one family, but the international impact of the new era.

In physiologic terms, the change Jean Pierre describes "I can now play with my friends" was due to changes in the circulation with exercise produced by the new anastomosis, or systemic to pulmonary shunt. Prior to the shunt, the child with tetralogy seeking the requisite increase in pulmonary blood flow on exercise was frustrated by the fixed obstruction of the pulmonary stenosis. After the shunt, as cardiac output increased, the obstruction was bypassed, and increased flow from the over-riding aorta passed down the subclavian artery to the lungs. This change in exercise tolerance was the greatest single benefit of the new operation to patients and families alike.

After the Blalock Taussig Shunt A year later, in 1945, Crafoord and Nylin of Stockholm introduced resection and end-to-end anastomosis for the repair of coarctation of the aorta [104].

Just as Harvey's work was stimulated by his studies in Padua [19], and Mall had learned much in the laboratory of His in Germany [65], so did pediatric cardiology now become part of a vibrant international network. The new Blalock Taussig operation, the quintessential collaboration of pediatric cardiologist and surgeon, spread rapidly around the world, and ushered in an era of intensive study and analysis of the physiology of the congenitally abnormal heart.

Many surgical modifications of the Blalock Taussig operation were developed, most of them variants of the concept of systemic to pulmonary arterial shunts, or forms of venous bypass [105]. In London in 1948 Russell (later Sir Russell) Brock [106] successfully pioneered a different concept, direct transventricular relief of the pulmonary stenosis; he referred to a prior attempt by Doyen in Paris in 1913 [107], an attempt which failed because the pulmonary stenosis was infundibular rather than valvar.

TOOLS OF DIAGNOSIS

New and better surgery demanded more precise definition and diagnosis of the underlying cardiac defect. The armamentarium of the cardiologist rapidly expanded from the stethoscope, fluoroscope and 6 lead electrocardiogram, to vectorcardiogram, phonocardiogram and cardiac catheterisation [16,90,91,108].

Electrocardiography The history of how the electrocardiogram was first used by clinicians was rather different for pediatric cardiologists than for internists. As Fye has shown [11], Thomas Lewis, Sir James Mackenzie and others who applied Einthoven's discovery to patients in the early years of the 20th century were primarily drawn to the study of arrhythmias, and only later recognised how valuable a tool this was in the diagnosis of myocardial ischemia.

By contrast, in children the electrocardiogram was for many years primarily thought of as a tool for the recognition of certain specific malformations. Later, signs of atrial and ventricular hypertrophy were used to assess physiologic severity of a defect such as pulmonary valve stenosis. Although arrhythmias were recognised, they did not come under intensive pediatric study until the late 1970s and early 1980s. A brief account of this sequence is outlined in chapter 6.

Prior to 1940 most published electrocardiograms showed only 6 standard leads [2,109], but by the mid 1950s precordial leads [110] were in widespread use. The amplitude and configuration of the different components of the PQRST complex were established for various ages [111-113]. Most infants and young children were known to have a rightward QRS axis, and some studies evaluated the diagnostic significance of a leftward axis in a cyanotic child [114,115]. Such studies were given impetus by the new pathologic classification of tricuspid atresia described by Jesse Edwards in 1949 [116]. The Mayo clinic group, among their innumerable contributions, also clarified the electrocardiographic pattern of atrioventricular septal defects [117]. Sodi Pallares of Mexico City was the first to recognise the distinctive sequence of ventricular activation seen in tetralogy of Fallot [118]. This is by no means an exhaustive listing of how the electrocardiogram was being studied at the time, but an indication of the approaches used by clinicians.

It is difficult to convey accurately the overlapping nature of diagnosis and therapy in those early years. One example is the diagnosis and surgery for atrial septal defect. Even before the advent of cardiopulmonary bypass, surgical repair of secundum atrial septal defect was being undertaken with the help of hypothermia or an atrial well technique. The intracardiac operating time available was around ten minutes, quite adequate for suture repair of a typical secundum defect, but repair of an ostium primum was impossible. Almost every cardiac center using hypothermia made at least one erroneous preoperative decision on the exact status of the atrial septum, since the clinicophysiologic profile of partial forms of atrioventricular septal defect was being established simultaneously with new forms of surgery.

Cardiac Catheterisation and Angiocardiography. Clearly cardiac catheterisation laboratories added much completely new information on cardiac pressures and volumes, and on myocardial metabolism [16]. In our context, these new laboratories provided hemodynamic data on the malformations and diseases previously described in clinical and anatomic terms.

The monograph by Cournand and his associates written in 1949 [91] gives a particularly interesting picture of the careful meticulous approach used in the famous catheterisation laboratory at Bellevue Hospital. The pediatric cardiologist of the group, Janet Baldwin, supplied the clinical data including chest Xray and six lead electrocardiogram, and in each case detailed the additional information supplied by the new, invasive procedure of cardiac catheterisation. One of the children (Case 16) whose study they reported, had tetralogy of Fallot with a right aortic arch. After cardiac catheterisation had confirmed the clinical diagnosis, he was then sent from Bellevue Hospital in New York City to Baltimore for the new procedure of a Blalock Taussig shunt. Almost everything used in diagnosis and treatment of this child, who did well, was new and dramatic, with long term consequences as yet unknown.

At the time Bing and his colleagues were making their remarkable contributions to the physiologic understanding of cyanotic heart defects [16], the cardiac catheterisation laboratory at Johns Hopkins was far removed from the laboratory, controlled by radiologists, where angiocardiograms could be performed. A great deal of logistic and conceptual effort was needed, much of it undertaken in other countries, particularly in Sweden by Kjellberg and his associates, before the advent of the modern peditric catheterisation laboratory. Angiocardiography was pioneered by Castellanos and his associates in Cuba [7,119]. Robb and Steinberg had also introduced the technique in the United States in 1939, but angiocardiography did not come into widespread use until the late 1940's and early 1950's [14]. For the first time the interior structure of the heart could be visualised in a living child outside the operating room.

The gradual integration of catheterisation and angiography into one laboratory, the growth of cineangiography, and the steady improvement in catheter equipment, all epitomised refinements in the tools needed for intravascular study [14-16].

NEW SURGICAL CONCEPTS

Two of the new surgical approaches of the early 1950's owed much to the hemodynamic information coming from the catheterisation laboratory. These were the Blalock-Hanlon procedure and pulmonary artery banding.

The Blalock Hanlon Procedure, described in 1950 [120], was the first of a number of valiant but hazardous attempts to increase intracardiac mixing in complete transposition. Although the clinical diagnosis of transposition had been described by Taussig many years earlier [18], it is uncertain if the concept of the need for increased mixing was clearly established until after some of these infants had undergone cardiac catheterisation. It was appreciated early that infants who had an additional large defect, whether at the atrial, ventricular or ductal level, were less cyanotic and survived longer than those with an intact septum. The Blalock Hanlon procedure, the surgical creation of an atrial septal defect, was a highly innovative operation, and did save some infants. The surgical difficulties, combined with the severe hypoxia of the infants treated, made this operation and its many later variants, in general, an unsatisfactory form of palliation.

Pulmonary Artery Banding was introduced in 1952 [121], and is discussed further in chapter 7. The remarkable concept of Muller and Damman, that banding of the pulmonary artery might protect the pulmonary vascular bed from the effects of a massive left to right shunt, would have been impossible without the new insights into pressure flow relationships gained from the tool of cardiac catheterisation. The tools of chest Xray and fluoroscopy, so valuable in analysis of tetralogy and some other cyanotic malformations, were of limited use in these new concepts. The evolution of the concept of pulmonary vascular obstructive disease as a complication of pulmonary hypertension was an outgrowth of many studies by clinicians, physiologists, and pathologists.

THE CHANGING OF THE GUARD

Although closed heart operations continued, the reign of closed heart surgery ended in 1955. During the intervening decade from 1945 to 1955, surgery advanced rapidly, and many new tools and concepts were developed. Each new tool enlarged the physiologic understanding of the heart, and stimulated the growth of clinician-physiologist-surgeon teams which continue to this day in all centers to work with varying degrees of successful symbiosis. This **team concept** was as new and as enduring as the surgical advance from which it developed. From the outset the Mayo Clinic provided a paradigm of this concept, in the high quality of scholarship and patient care, collegial interaction, and durability of their team.

By the time the open heart era dawned, the physiology and anatomy of most cardiac defects could be clearly defined prior to surgery. Diagnosis was no longer dependent only on skilful building, or stitching together, of a clinical profile, but was subject to hemodynamic and angiographic confirmation. Even more importantly, the use of these new tools led to early studies of myocardial metabolism and an understanding of the physiology of both normal and abnormal hearts.

Preventive Cardiology

Risk factors for adult heart disease were coming under scrutiny [122] with the beginning of the Framingham study and with more widespread use of blood pressure measurements in children. However, during the exciting dawn of heart surgery, the focus was on clinical diagnosis, physiology and treatment of defects, and preventive cardiology had not yet emerged as a major area of interest for pediatricians.

The Child with Heart Disease

Publication of the new treatment for cyanotic children came at the end of the second World War. Communications and travel between medical centers was again possible, and the good news travelled fast. The child with heart disease was now potentially treatable, and became a subject for discussion in the lay Press. Helen Taussig told how parents would bring a cyanotic child from a long distance, after they had discussed the symptoms with neighbors or friends. She maintained that squatting when tired was common in older children with tetralogy of Fallot, and that several parents had told her they had felt hopeful and ready to come, once they knew their child had this symptom in common with another child who had undergone a successful shunt procedure.

In some respects the growth of pediatric cardiology from clinics devoted to rheumatic fever was helpful. Long term follow up was an integral part of such clinics, and even in the strenuous early years Taussig and other pioneers arranged for sequential visits for children who had undergone surgery, and also for others for whom no operation could yet be done. The 1940s and early 1950s saw not only the dawn of heart surgery, but the advent of penicillin and the antibiotic era. The future seemed extraordinarily bright, even though open heart surgery was not yet available.

ADDITIONAL REFERENCES AND NOTES

84. Gross RE, Hubbard JP. Surgical ligation of a patent ductus arteriosus: Report of first successful case. JAMA 1939;112:729-731.

85. Brieger GH. The development of surgery. In: Sabiston DC, editor. Textbook of surgery 14th ed. Philadelphia: Saunders, 1991:1-18.

86. Ravitch MM. Alfred Blalock 1889-1964. Baltimore: Johns Hopkins Press, 1966.

87. Longmire WP Jr. Alfred Blalock. His Life and Times. WP Longmire 1991.

88. Glenn WWL. The Development of Cardiac Surgery 1896-1991 Permanent exhibit in Cushing Library Yale University from 1992.

89. Bing RJ, Vandam LD, Gray FD Jr. Physiologic studies in congenital heart disease. I. Procedures. Bull Johns Hopkins Hosp 1947; 80:107-120.

90. Dexter LFW, Haynes CS, Burwell EC, Eppinger R, Siebel D, Evans JN. Studies of congenital heart disease.J Clin Inv 1947;26: 547-576.

91. Cournand A, Baldwin JS, Himmelstein A. Cardiac Catheterisation in Congenital Heart Disease: A Clinical and Physiologic Study in Infants and Children. New York, Commonwealth Fund 1949.

92. Barclay AE, Barcroft SJ, Barron DH, Franklin KJ. A radiographic demonstration of the circulation through the heart in the adult and in the fetus, and the identification of the ductus arteriosus. Brit J Radiol 1939;12:505-517.

93. Civin WH, Edwards JE. The postnatal structural changes in the intrapulmonary arteries and arterioles. Arch Path 1951;51:192-200.

94. James LS, Rowe RD. The pattern of response of pulmonary and systemic arterial pressures in newborn and older infants to short periods of hypoxia. J Pediatrics 1957;51:5-11.

95. Neill CA. Development of the pulmonary veins. With reference to anomalies of the pulmonary venous return. Pediatrics 1956;18:880-887.

96. Paget S. Surgery of the Chest. London, John Wright 1896:121.

97. Rehn L. Ueber penetrierende Hertzwundenund Herznaht. Arch Klin Chir 1897;55:315.

98. Levy SE, Blalock A.. Experimental observations on the effects of connecting by suture the left main pulmonary artery to the systemic circulation. J Thorac Surg 1939;8:525-528.

99. Thomas VT. Pioneering Research in Surgical Shock and Cardiovascular Surgery. Vivien Thomas and His Work with Alfred Blalock. An Autobiography by Vivien T.Thomas. Philadelphia, U Pennsylvania Press, 1985.

100. Blalock A, Taussig HB. Surgical treatment of malformations of the heart; in which there is pulmonary stenosis or pulmonary atresia. JAMA 1945; 128:189-202.

101. Whittemore R. Interview in The Hopkins Advocate 1994;11:issue 1,1-3.

102. Whittemore R, Hobbins JC, Engle MA. Pregnancy and its outcome in women with and without surgical treatment of congenital heart disease. Am J Cardiol 1982;50:641-651.

103. Bahnson HT. Classics in thoracic surgery: Surgical treatment of pulmonic stenosis: a retrospection. Ann Thorac Surg 1982;33:96-98.

104. Crafoord C, Nylin G. Congenital coarctation of the aorta and its surgical treatment. J Thorac Surg 1945;14:347-361.

105. Glenn WWL, Palino JF. Circulatory bypass of the right heart. I. Preliminary observation on direct delivery of vena caval blood in pulmonary arterial circulation. Azygos vein pulmonary artery shunt. Yale J Biol Med 1954;27:147-151.

106. Brock RC. Pulmonary valvulotomy for the relief of congenital pulmonary stenosis. Report of three cases. Brit Med J 1948;1:1121-1126.

107. Doyen E. Brief communication. Presse medicale 1913;21:860.

108. Swan HJC, Hetzel PS, Wood EH. Quantitative estimation by indicator-dilution techniques of contribution of blood to the left-to-right shunt in atrial septal defect. Circulation 1956;14:212-220.

109. Schnitker MA. The electrocardiogram in congenital heart disease. (A study of 109 cases, 106 withautopsy). Cambridge: Harvard University Press, 1940.

110. Wilson FN, Johnston FD, Rosenbaum FF, Barker PS. On Einthoven's triangle, the theory of unipolarelectrocardiographic leads, and the interpretation of the precordial electrocardiogram. Am Heart J 1946;32:277-310.

111. Ziegler RF. Electrocardiographic studies in normal infants and children. Springfield, Charles C Thomas, 1951.

112. Yu PNG, Joos HA, Katsampes CP. Unipolar electrocardiograms in normal infants and children. Am Heart J 1951;41:91-104.

113. Burch GE, De Pasquale NP. A history of electrocardiography. Chicago, Year Book Publishers 1964.

114. Donzelot E, Durand M, Metianu C, Vlad P. L'axe electrique normal ou devie a gauche dans les cardiopathies congenitales cyanogenes. Etude de 29 personnel interet diagnostique. Arch mal coeur 1950;43:577-582.

115. Neill CA, Brink AJ. Left axis deviation in tricuspid atresia and single ventricle: The electrocardiogram in 36 autopsied cases. Circulation 1955;12:612-619.

116. Edwards JE, Burchell HB. Congenital tricuspid atresia: A classification. Med Clin N America 1949;33:1177-1181.

117. Toscano-Barbosa E, Brandenburg RU, Burchell HB. Electrocardiographic studies of cases with intracardiac malformations of the atrioventricular canal. Proc Staff Meetings Mayo Clinic 1956;31:513-523.

118. Sodi-Pallares D. New bases of electrocardiography. St Louis, Mosby 1956.

119. Castellanos A, Pereiras R, Garcia A. La Angio-Cardiografia en el Nino: Angiocardiography in the Child. 7th Congress Pan American Medical Association, Havana 1939.

120. Blalock A, Hanlon CR. The surgical treatment of complete transposition of the aorta and pulmonary artery. Surg Gyn Obstet 1950; 90:1-15.

121. Muller WH, Damman JF. The treatment of certain congenital malformations of the heart by the creation of pulmonic stenosis to reduce pulmonary hypertension and excessive pulmonary blood flow. Surg Gyn Obstet 1952;95:213-219.

122. Keys A. Prediction and possible prevention of coronary heart disease. Am J Pub Health 1953;43:1399-1407.

CHAPTER 5

Open Heart Surgery 1955–mid 1970s

- Cardiopulmonary bypass: concepts and tools
- Surgical advances, new pathologic insights (conducting system, other)
- Rashkind balloon atrial septostomy
- Rheumatic heart disease
- Mitral valve prolapse
- The pioneer patient

Introduction

Today, in the 1990s, the greatest volume of both cardiac surgery and interventional cardiology is performed in adults with acquired heart disease, especially that due to coronary atherosclerosis. It is sometimes forgotten that the pioneering efforts of both open heart surgery and interventional catheterisation began with children. Just as closed heart surgery for children ushered in the dawn of therapy, so did cardiopulmonary bypass begin with the young. For both children and adults with heart disease, cardiopulmonary bypass and Rashkind's balloon atrial septostomy were the crowning achievements of the two decades from 1955 to the mid 1970s.

During the period open repair of cardiac anomalies became feasible there was a rapid emergence of new knowledge in all 4 domains of pediatric cardiology. The use of cardiopulmonary bypass enlarged the scope of research questions, and added new members to the cardiac teams involved in patient care. The nature and importance of pulsatile flow, the optimal way to protect the myocardium during surgery, methods for averting cerebral complications, were all new questions.

Most of the work on these issues was undertaken by surgeons and their associates. Nevertheless, pediatric cardiology was profoundly affected by the new methods. Preoperative evaluation and postoperative care assumed new dimensions. Now that the heart was being opened, the exact details of intracardiac anatomy needed to be known preoperatively. Anatomic precision was a stringent requirement. It was not enough to know that the patient had tetralogy, but the size and structure of the pulmonary artery branches was much more significant than in the past. To take another very simple example, the unexpected finding of a left superior vena cava was a minor affair during closed heart surgery, but might interfere with cardiopulmonary bypass in troublesome ways when all the techniques were new.

Second, the postoperative findings and complications were different and more complex. A child who had had an excellent open repair of tetralogy had residual murmurs of mild residual pulmonary stenosis and insufficiency, and right bundle branch block on the electrocardiogram. The long term significance of these changes and the likelihood of their progression was as yet unknown. Other new problems, heart block, post pericardiotomy syndrome, hemolysis, and late onset arrhythmias were all unexpected and unwelcome developments. Even more dreaded was the rare sequel of profound neurologic impairment. Immediate postoperative monitoring became more intensive, ultimately requiring new team members skilled in anaesthesia and respiratory management.

Above all, this was a period of excitement and innovation. Heart surgery was now envisioned as curative, rather than palliative. There seemed no limit to what would soon be accomplished.

In this more complex era, the collaborative team approach became even more critical than in past years. Surgical skill remained paramount, but much new help was needed from pathology, physiology, and skilled angiography. The caliber and sophistication of the bypass or pump team, the anaesthetists, and those monitoring in intensive care all played a role in establishing a successful new type of cardiac program.

THE OPEN HEART

The heart could now be opened, but pediatric cardiology was by no means yet an open book.

In this chapter we will discuss open heart surgery rather briefly. There is a plethora of excellent textbooks and papers on the subject [12,13]. Instead we will focus on how this surgery produced major changes in pediatric cardiology during the two decades from 1955 to the mid-1970s. Now that the heart could be opened and intracardiac defects closed, a new series of questions arose, questions not addressed in the closed heart era, when most of the patients were severely cyanotic or in heart failure. The question, did every defect need to be closed, stimulated studies of "Natural history." Since it was clearly impossible to withold life saving surgery from a child with a large ventricular septal defect, such studies included both operated and unoperated patients, the natural and unnatural history, as it was termed.

Some of the surgical findings stimulated clinicians and laboratory teams to more meticulous preoperative studies; such findings included the freqency of partial anomalous pulmonary venous drainage in atrial septal defect, the many variations in anatomy of ventricular septal defect, and coronary artery variations in tetralogy of Fallot. Postoperative complications stimulated new interest in electrophysiology, which became a major subject of study in the infant era beginning in the mid 1970s.

OTHER HEART PROBLEMS

In addition to discussing the impact of Rashkind's balloon atrial septostomy, we will also give an overview in this chapter of how rheumatic fever and mitral valve prolapse changed during these twenty years. One of the major developments was the growth of physiologic research concentrating on the young heart, and the concurrent growth of clinical studies documenting the challenge of heart disease in infancy.

The Normal Heart and Circulation

Pediatric cardiology expanded from clinical diagnosis to a search for deeper understanding of how the fetal and neonatal heart differed from that of the adult. The pioneering studies of Barclay [92] on the fetal circulation in animals had led to recognition that this was a fruitful area for pediatric research. The physiology of neonatal and fetal animals was under active investigation in the two decades from the mid 1950s to mid 1970s. New young investigators, not content only with descriptive diagnosis, now began to study with one of the few teams of neonatal physiologists, and then established laboratories of their own. These laboratories not only yielded new research knowledge on the perinatal heart and circulation, but provided useful physiologic training and concepts for new Fellows entering the field of pediatric cardiology.

Cardiac catheterisation in human infants began to be successfully performed in many centers, especially in divisions of cardiology which formed part of large childrens hospitals, such as Great Ormond Street Hospital in London or the Hospital for Sick Children in Toronto. Although almost all of these studies were performed in sick infants with highly complex intracardiac defects [123], the findings emphasised the need for further laboratory investigations of cardiopulmonary changes in the perinatal period.

The ductus arteriosus could now be visualised angiographically in the human newborn, and in the fetal animal. This visualisation, and new techniques of fetal research, led to much clinical study of the mechanisms and timing of normal ductal closure, a subject which continued a focus of research by Richard Rowe throughout his lifetime. Rudolph and his group embarked on many decades of innovative study of the circulation and hemodynamics of the fetal lamb [124]. The interrelationship of neonatal physiology with changes in the pulmonary vascular bed, begun in the 1950s, continued to be studied [125]. New tools were used to compare the innervation of immature and adult myocardium [126].

Thus in the two decades preceding successful therapy in infants, the infant era, a new body of knowledge was being developed on how the fetal and newborn heart differed from that of the mature individual. This body of knowledge eventually and laboriously came to be applied in patient care, both on the wards and in intensive care settings. The advances in fetal and neonatal physiology depended on the innovative minds of investigators, helped by new investigative tools, such as microcatheters.

The Developing Heart

Cardiac development became a focus of intensive research during the decades of the 50s and 60s. Many of these contributions were reviewed by van Mierop in 1979 [61]. The concept of staging of embryonic development allowed for the graphic depiction of simultaneous growth of the heart and other organs. This staging concept came into widespread use among clinicians and neonatologists seeking for an embryologic background for common childhood syndromes [127,127a].

EXPERIMENTAL EMBRYOLOGY

Technical laboratory advances had increased the scope of experimental embryology, which was now more widely used. A number of new concepts evolved from this work, including the importance of cell migration, and the interaction of form and function in the developing heart.

Radionuclide labelling began to be used by Rosenquist [128] and others to document the origin of cells which migrated into various areas of the embryo heart. These studies, later supplemented by experiments with chimera preparations, contributed to a number of later discoveries, such as the role of neural crest cells in aortopulmonary septation.

Electron microscopy studies, especially those of Tomas Pexieder of Lausanne [129], provided exquisite detailed information on the growth of the ventricular septum, and the formation of the right ventricular outflow tract.

Rychter demonstrated that a variety of intracardiac malformations could be induced by constricting the aortic arches in the embryonic chick heart [130]. Later experiments by Clark and associates inducing alterations in embryonic flows and pressures [131] brought to life an important new concept, the continuing **interaction of form and function** in the embryonic heart.

Experimental teratology was not a new concept, for numerous attempts to induce major anomalies in laboratory animals had been made since the 1930s. Josef Warkany and his colleagues in Cincinnatti had begun the new field of cardiovascular teratogenesis in the mid 1940s by producing aortic arch and cardiac anomalies in the offspring of Vitamin A deficient rats [132]. In the 1960s the possible role of teratogens in cardiac defects came under study both in the laboratory and in human populations.

TERATOLOGY

The concept that cardiovascular malformations could be chemically induced using the tools of experimental teratology was pioneered in the 1950s [133,134]. Fox and Goss [133] showed that complete transposition could be produced in the offspring of experimental animals by the injection of trypan blue at a specific time in pregnancy. This work aroused great hopes that the basic mechanism of this severe defect would soon be understood, a hope which has not yet been completely realised.

Embryopathy in the Human Fetus. Interest in environmental teratogenesis was further aroused by the major pandemics of rubella embryopathy which occurred twenty years apart, in the early 1940s and early 1960s [135,136]. The combination of patent ductus and peripheral pulmonic stenosis, so characteristic of rubella embryopathy, was compatible with viral invasion and damage to the fourth and sixth aortic arches on the surface of the embryo, analogous to the invasion of the lens of the eye, the otic capsule, and the brain. The epidemics led to much experimental effort to induce cardiac defects with viral infections, and to some early epidemiologic approaches seeking to correlate human cardiac defects with other maternal illness, including mumps. None of these efforts led to conclusive evidence implicating any virus other than rubella as a cardiac teratogen in humans.

Thalidomide: During the 1960s two other events led to an great resurgence of interest in cardiac teratogenesis in humans. One was thalidomide embryopathy, the outbreak of phocomelia and cardiac anomalies attributable to maternal thalidomide ingestion at a sensitive period in pregnancy. This epidemic affected mainly West Germany, where the drug was manufactured, but also a number of infants in Canada, Australia and the British Isles. The drug had not been licensed in the United States, and thus only a few sporadic cases occurred. The other event which stimulated the search for human cardiac teratogens was the definition of Williams syndrome, in which cardiovascular defects, especially supravalvar aortic and pulmonic stenosis, were combined with features of infantile hypercalcemia.

Although the most dramatic and devastating feature of thalidomide embryopathy was phocomelia [137-140], about one fifth of all affected infants had cardiac defects, often tetralogy of Fallot with extreme pulmonic stenosis or atresia. Two decades later many of the cardiac features of retinoic acid embryopathy were found to be similar [141]. The public health impact of the thalidomide embryopathy was enormous, resulting in greatly increased powers and visibility for the Federal Drug Administration, and an intense research effort on teratogenesis in animals. Thalidomide itself, however, did not prove a useful drug in inducing cardiac anomalies experimentally.

Williams-Beuren Syndrome: A "flurry of interest" in the possible role of abnormal Vitamin D metabolism followed the first descriptions of supravalvar aortic stenosis in the Williams-Beuren syndrome [142-144]. The recognition of the syndrome led to increased attention to the concept of genetic environmental interaction in cardiac maldevelopment. The clinical photograph in Williams original paper of the four children with similar facies is perhaps one of the most often reproduced of all such group pictures in pediatric cardiology. Black and Bonham Carter in London drew attention to the possible overlap of the syndrome with infantile hypercalcemia.

Some features of supravalvar aortic stenosis were reproduced experimentally in rabbits. A pediatric literature grew on the "elfin facies," the cocktail party manner, and the facial changes with aging. Alois Beuren in Göttingen, Germany collected a large group of photographs from his own clinical experience, covering the door inside his office. At that time it was the custom to administer a large dose of Vitamin D intramuscularly to pregnant mothers in West Germany, and the question arose if the German experience of a large number of cases was related to this super efficient method of preventing infantile rickets.

By the mid 1960s it seemed quite clear that there were two etiologies for supravalvar aortic stenosis. It could occur as a rare familial cardiac defect inherited as an autosomal dominant; or be sporadic, associated with mental retardation, infantile hypercalcemia and multiple extracardiac defects—the Williams-Beuren syndrome. This clear cut separation was challenged shortly thereafter. It now appears as if both forms of the disorder are due to a defect in the elastin gene [145]. Elucidation of how the two forms are related is still under study.

The demonstrated vulnerability of the heart to environmental agents led to the search for other potential teratogens [146]. Sheila Mitchell reviewed the data from the massive collaborative perinatal study, and compared the pregnancy experience of mothers of children born with heart defects to those with normal hearts. Maternal diabetes was clearly implicated as increasing the risk of a heart defect; the possible implication of a number of medications, including maternal hormone ingestion, emphasised the need for further epidemiologic approaches.

GENETICS AND ENVIRONMENT

Research into possible genetic mechanisms of cardiac defects by now included some of the early clinical family studies [147,148]. Donald Patterson, recognising the predisposition of certain breeds of dogs to distinctive cardiac malformations, began a series of inbreeding experiments which contributed greatly to genetic knowledge. His early studies on patent ductus [149] showed conclusively that repeated inbreeding resulted in an extremely high incidence of the defect; of even more interest, he was able to show that some of the offspring who did not have a clinically apparent patent duct, had a large ductus diverticulum on aortography. This introduced the concept that a "forme fruste," or clinically inapparent form of a cardiac defect, might be present in relatives of affected children. The new tools of echocardiography and molecular biology are now making it possible to explore this concept in human populations.

Chromosomal anomalies: Two important discoveries were made during this time, both concerning the genetics of atrioventricular septal defect. One was a clinical study of Down syndrome, the other, with even wider implications, was the harbinger of the future application of molecular biologic techniques to pediatric cardiology.

In 1961 Rowe and Uchida [150], in a meticulous clinical study of a population of infants with Down syndrome, established the extraordinarily high prevalence of congenital heart defects (40%); they also confirmed an unusual distribution of defects, including the predominance of atrioventricular and other septal defects, and the absence of transposition or anomalies of cardiac looping. Although Abbott had already commented on the association of Down syndrome and defects in atrioventricular septation, the literature prior to Rowe and Uchida was confusing, since the distribution of cardiac anomalies was different in different age groups. Rowe and Uchida obtained as close as possible to a birth sample, by studying young infants referred for dermatoglyphic analysis to confirm the clinical diagnosis of Down syndrome.

Lejeune's discovery of the chromosomal basis of Down syndrome, reported in 1959 [151], opened a new field of study into the multihandicapped child. The full implications of both these discoveries are only now, almost forty years later, being fully recognised.

Cardiac Defects and Childhood Heart Disease

By 1955 pediatric cardiac units were present in most major children's centers around the world, and the numbers continued to grow rapidly over the next twenty years. Advances were made in the recognition of myocardial disorders [152,153], infective endocarditis [154] and pediatric arrhythmias [155]. Kawasaki disease was described in Japan in 1967 [156], but did not become recognised as a significant problem in the West until almost a decade later. Mitral valve prolapse was defined [157], and rheumatic fever was showing a changing pattern, discussed in a monograph by Milton Markowitz and Anne Kuttner [158].

In this rapidly expanding age of pediatric cardiology, the most explosive changes continued to occur in congenital heart disease, both in the understanding of clinicophysiologic concepts, and in the beginning of open heart surgery.

OPEN HEART SURGERY

A few centers had undertaken closure of atrial septal defects of the secundum type using whole body cooling in the early 1950's [159]. Wilfred Bigelow of Toronto has described some of the early history of his own pioneering work with this technique in a monograph combining scientific information, clarity and humor in model proportions [160]. The title is "Cold Hearts," but the book has a warm sense of collegiality, and pays tribute to the new breed of technicians and research associates entering research laboratories and the clinical arena. Transventricular relief of pulmonary valve stenosis had also been successful by use of this technique.

However, open heart surgery in the modern sense is usually dated to 1955. Successful intracardiac repair of ventricular septal defects and tetralogy of Fallot began in Minneapolis when Walton Lillehei and associates in 1955 used human cross circulation techniques [161]. This feat was both admired and censured at the time, because of the possible risk to the healthy parent. Lillehei and his group shortly thereafter changed to the use of cardiopulmonary bypass, and continued for many years to be leaders in open heart surgery. At a medical meeting at Howard University in the late 1980's Lillehei described how as a very young man he had watched the inexorable death from heart failure of a seventeen year old girl with an atrial septal defect. Seeing the simplicity of the defect at autopsy was an inspiration to him to persevere in the search for a cure.

Cardiopulmonary Bypass: The essential tool of an effective mechanical form of cardiopulmonary bypass is owed to John H. Gibbon Jr. of Philadelphia [162]. The concept of extracorporeal circulatory support already existed; some of its history is reviewed in surgical textbooks [12,13], and by Hewitt & Creech [163]. Shumacker [12] describes Gibbon's work and some of the later modifications in detail, and gives an absorbing account of a number of earlier efforts to maintain perfusion of the brain and vital organs while the heart was open.

The modified Gibbon pump was used by Kirklin and his group at the Mayo clinic in 1955 in their original series of intracardiac repairs using cardiopulmonary bypass [164]. All those whose names are listed on this original paper contributed much to pediatric cardiology; Jim DuShane was for many years the chief of pediatric cardiology at the Mayo Clinic, and played a major role in defining the clinical specialty; Earl Wood's laboratory produced new physiologic information of unrivalled quality. John Kirklin's contributions to the growth and improvement of heart surgery in children have been legendary, both during his years at the Mayo Clinic, and later at the University of Alabama.

Pediatric Cardiology and the Rise of Open Heart Surgery. Quite suddenly, a whole new group of children had entered the realm of treatment. The indications for treatment were often less well defined than in the prior era of closed heart surgery. For every patient with an atrial septal defect who was in heart failure, and clearly needed help, there were perhaps a hundred who were leading normal lives. They were quite unlike the cyanotic children who poured into heart centers in the late 1940s and early 1950s. Fortunately, the early surgical results with atrial defect repair were highly encouraging, even outside the major regional centers.

With more complex defects, a tension began, one which was not resolved till the onset of the infant era. The tension was due to the fact that the sickest children were the youngest, and had the most complex defects. Yet it soon became apparent that cardiopulmonary bypass was still hazardous in most young infants. This tension was perhaps best exemplified by complete atrioventricular septal defect. With few exceptions, attempts to repair such defects in the early years of open heart surgery resulted in high rates of mortality and morbidity. Some groups favored banding in infancy, with later repair; others felt banding increased the hazards of later operation. Yet without banding, such patients rapidly developed pulmonary vascular obstructive disease.

Advances were slowed by the complication of heart block, which in turn led to further study of the conducting system in both normal and malformed hearts. Maurice Lev of Chicago was a leader among cardiac pathologists in redefining the site of the atrioventricular node and the course of the right and left bundle branches [165]. New pathologic insights were provided during these years into well established cardiac problems. The concept of Grover Hutchins that coarctation of the aorta represented a branch point of the ductus arteriosus [166] helped draw attention to coarctation as part of a spectrum of defects involved in disturbances of intrauterine left heart flow [131]; his study and others emerging from laboratories of fetal research, focussed surgical attention on the important role of ductal tissue in coarctation, which was no longer a simple "shelf." Bill Roberts' convincing demonstration that isolated aortic stenosis, even late in life when the valve was calcified, represented a congenital defect, brought insight into the spectrum of severity of congenital malformations [167].

This period was characterised by a great increase in the number of therapeutic centers, and by the formation of interdisciplinary groups to study the new problems raised by advancing knowledge. Inadequate methods of myocardial preservation, and problems with controlling bleeding from collateral arteries in cyanotic adults were among many other new problems encountered.

Controversy arose over the indications and timing of open repair, particularly of ventricular septal defects. The concept of prognosis, or natural history, was not new, being mentioned in the mid 19th century by Peacock [10], and studied more recently by others [168,169]. Spontaneous closure of ventricular septal defects had been documented [170], but there were many gaps in knowledge. Some of these were addressed by the Natural History Study [171] of over 2,000 medically and surgically treated children with ventricular septal defect, pulmonary stenosis or aortic stenosis, one of the earliest collaborative large scale clinical trials in cardiology. This study makes interesting reading even today, showing the methods used at the time to correlate clinical findings and defect severity, and some of the postoperative progress of the patients followed.

After Open Repair? Methods to improve the completeness and accuracy of diagnosis continued to be described in these two decades. Postoperative changes became a major focus of pediatric cardiologists, and a number of symposia and publications resulted.

Morriss and McNamara [172] wrote a much quoted chapter on "Residua, sequelae and complications of surgery for congenital heart disease." They defined residua as problems remaining from the original defect, such as a small residual shunt across the septum after surgical closure of a ventricular septal defect. Sequelae were results of the surgery, such as the right bundle branch block so frequent after tetralogy repair. Complications they defined as unexpected events, such as injury to the phrenic nerve, mediastinitis, or arrhythmias. Despite the many subsequent papers on the topic of postoperative evaluation, pediatric cardiologists and surgeons never reached a consensus on how best to present the data. Many surgical papers use mortality, freedom from reoperation, and pressure gradients as yardsticks: only recently have considerations of quality of life entered this important area of study. In the same volume as Morriss and McNamara's discussion, Keane and associates [172a] describe noninvasive techniques in postoperative assessment, one of the earliest accounts of the beginning role of echocardiography in this field. The volume as a whole, published in 1975, provides a good outline of the status of postoperative study immediately before the dawn of the infant era.

Complete Transposition New tools and concepts allowed surgeons to intervene succesfully on complex and previously lethal defects, including complete transposition [173,174]. It is difficult for a non-surgeon to understand why Senning's operation of intra-atrial switching for transposition did not "catch on" in 1959, but returned to international favor twenty years later, only to be replaced by Jatene's arterial switch.

Bill Mustard, working at the Hospital for Sick Children in Toronto, was alerted by John Keith to the tragic number of early infant deaths attributable to transposition. These infants not only died very early, within the first month or two of life, but they were also singularly free of chromosomal or other extracardiac defects, thus compounding the tragedy of their loss. Mustard was fascinated by transpositon; as early as 1952, long before cardiopulmonary bypass, he attempted a switch procedure on an infant using a monkey lung for oxygenation. The monkey lung filled inexorably with edema fluid faster than surgery could be completed. This harrowing attempt thus preceded his triumphant account of the new Mustard operation by twelve long years. Once cardiopulmonary bypass techniques became established, he continued to work on the intricacies of an intra-atrial baffle. Although his colleagues, Keith, Vlad and Rowe, later joined by Langford Kidd, were highly adept at early and correct diagnosis, the risks of anesthesia and surgery in neonates were still high; several of Mustard's early successes were in infants or even young children over six months of age, who had somehow survived the neonatal period. (A few had first undergone a Blalock Hanlon procedure as neonates, but this operation always remained hazardous, without an appreciable learning curve. Other attempts to increase intracardiac mixing, such as the Baffes procedure, while successful in Chicago, proved resistant to export). Fortunately, only two years after surgeons around the world started learning how to perform the Mustard operation [174], the prognosis of the neonate with transposition was transformed by the birth of invasive cardiology. In 1966 William Rashkind of Philadelphia introduced the therapeutic balloon catheter.

RASHKIND'S BALLOON ATRIAL SEPTOSTOMY

The use of a balloon catheter to increase cardiac mixing in transposition [175] is a good example of the interaction of tools and concepts. Baillie, in the 18th century, had been the first to comment on the lack of mixing of the "florid" blood with the dark or venous blood in this "singular malformation" [43a]. The concept that increased cardiac mixing at the atrial level could improve cyanosis in transposition dated back to the first successful atrial septectomy by Blalock and Hanlon in 1950 [120]. Vivien Thomas [99] gives an absorbing account of the laborious development of this procedure, including the search for the optimal tool or instrument.

Two hundred years after Baillie and almost twenty years after Blalock and Hanlon, Rashkind articulated the concept that intracardiac mixing must be increased in the **neonate**, since most deaths occurred early; that for this purpose, the surgeon's knife could and should be replaced; and he developed the necessary tool, the balloon catheter which started the whole brilliant expanding field of **interventional cardiology**. The growth of interventional cardiology is discussed further in chapter 6.

Dan McNamara of Houston, a long time friend of Rashkind, described his balloon atrial septostomy as one of the most important therapeutic procedures of the quarter century between 1958 and 1983 [176]. After analysing its importance, he writes:

> *"The dexterous Rashkind had not appreciated that the procedure might be less successful in other cardiologists hands. Rashkind had taught that rapid withdrawal across the foramen ovale of the fully inflated balloon was important, but he insisted that the procedure is actually very simple: 'All it requires is a big jerk on the end of the catheter . . .' Rashkind would quip whenever he was invited to speak on his method. It was partly Rashkind's humorous and entertaining manner of speaking, his enthusiasm for teaching and his interest in travel that took him to virtually every major city in most countries of the world to tell about the balloon catheter and the whole subject of transposition . . ."*

At a meeting held in 1994 to dedicate the Rashkind research chair of pediatric cardiology at Childrens Hospital of Philadelphia, several of the speakers gathered to pay posthumous tribute repeated Bill Rashkind's quip. It was greeted with gentle and nostalgic laughter by the large audience of former colleagues, patients and donors who remembered him, as Dan McNamara describes him, an energetic pioneer, a great and lovable man who combined clinical and technical skill with historical scholarship [7,24] and empathy. Tsung Cheng, in the introduction to his book on valvuloplasty [177] reproduces the page from JAMA where Rashkind and Miller's paper originally appeared; he notes that a typing error in the legend describing the illustration of Rashkind's catheter had changed the word "magnified" to "magnificent." It is probably one of the few occasions in medical writing where a typo was ahead of later eloquence.

CONGENITAL DEFECTS: MEDICAL AND SURGICAL ADVANCES

Homografts [178], conduits [179] and electronic pacemakers [180,181] were introduced for pediatric patients. Rastelli and his colleagues at the Mayo Clinic in 1968 [182] modified the surgical approach to the atrioventricular valve in atrioventricular septal defects, thus transforming the outcome of repair of this treacherous and anatomically variable defect.

The 1970s saw the development of surgical treatment of highly complex defects [183], and increasing sophistication in the use of diagnostic tools, including the electrocardiogram and angiocardiogram [184-7]. These advances in precision and quantitation, coming from many different geographic centers, were leading pediatric cardiology toward the infant era.

Early Diagnosis and Referral became an increasing focus of pediatric cardiology as new therapies became more successful. A number of efforts began to build efficient referral networks, and to increase collaboration between cardiologists, neonatologists and pediatricians [176]. The paradigm of this effort was provided by Don Fyler and his colleagues of the **New England Regional Infant Cardiac Program**. Their study and program, a truly remarkable and perhaps unrivalled combination of "outreach," patient care, and research, was begun in 1968, and the major analysis was for the years 1968-1974. Although their full report was not issued until 1980 [188], the widespread knowledge and interim reports of their work was vital in focusing attention on the benefits of regionalised care. By their careful analysis of both cardiac and extracardiac problems in infants hospitalised under one year of age they provided a vivid picture of the status of the infant in the open heart era, before open heart repair in infancy for most defects became the norm.

RHEUMATIC FEVER AND RHEUMATIC HEART DISEASE

Worldwide, rheumatic heart disease does not fit neatly into any era. Like the poor, it is always with us, yet it is now seldom seen in developed countries. Lewis and Gotsman [189] describe the natural history of rheumatic heart disease in childhood under 4 headings: 1) as seen in the United States and Great Britain in the decades 1930-1950, before the era of antibiotics and antiinflammatory agents: 2) the modification of the disease by effective management of streptococcal infections and vigorous management of acute attacks: 3) the residual scourge that occurs in poor countries or underprivileged or developing countries where chemoprophylaxis and effective therapy are not available: 4) the natural history of chronic established rheumatic valve disease.

We have elected to discuss childhood rheumatic heart problems very briefly here, using 1965 to symbolise a watershed year, a time when the disease had already changed dramatically. Sydenham's chorea, the Carey Coomb's murmur, and rheumatic nodules were beginning to pass into the medical history of the Western world. Markowitz and Kuttner, in the preface to their monograph on rheumatic fever in 1965 [158], wrote of the already changing pattern and decline of a once dreaded disease. They quoted from a lecture by Cheadle given in 1888:

> *"there is perhaps no serious disease more familiar to us than acute articular rheumatism; it is one of the disorders most commonly seen in the wards of a general hospital; it is constantly encountered in private practice ..."*

They then quoted from Glover, who noted in 1930 that the incidence of acute rheumatism was slowly but surely declining, but "we are still painfully aware of those many patients who, in what should be their happy youth or vigorous manhood, perish slowly of rheumatic heart disease."

Markowitz and Kuttner attributed the changes between 1888 and 1930 to improved social conditions. Milton Markowitz, now emeritus Dean for students at Hartford Connecticut, had trained as a pediatrician; in 1965 he was chief of pediatrics at Sinai Hospital in Baltimore, and had succeeded Helen Taussig as Director of the rheumatic fever clinic at Johns Hopkins. Anne Kuttner had started as a Ph.D. bacteriologist at the Rockefeller Institute, with a special interest in the streptococcus, and after obtaining her M.D degree studied rheumatic fever in New York, in Peiping China, and at Irvington House, the convalescent home for rheumatic fever for New York City. Until the late 1960's there was a similar convalescent home in most major cities in the USA, all of which are now used for other purposes. Many of the major studies which documented the continuing changing pattern of rheumatic fever came from follow up of children who had been in such homes in Boston, Chicago and elsewhere. It is not possible to do justice to these contributions in this brief section, but the names of many of the researchers are among the great pioneers of those who worked for heart health in children.

The two authors note that between 1930 and the mid 1960s the disease continued to decline, both in incidence and severity. Studies in Denmark had documented a fall in the attack rate of acute rheumatic fever in young children from 45/10,000 in 1885 to 5/10,000 in 1945. Markowitz and Kuttner postulated that some of the continuing decline between 1930 and the mid 1960s could have been due to the introduction of antibiotics, with vigorous treatment of Group A streptococcal infections; some to more aggressive management of any acute episode of rheumatic fever with salicylates or steroids. Secondary prophylaxis, which had begun in the 1940's with sulfanilamide [190], was now being administered as penicillin, either orally in daily doses or by monthly intramuscular injection. Their monograph is an excellent resource for the earlier literature in the field, and a complete summary of then current knowledge of the role of the streptococcus and the clinical manifestations of rheumatic fever and carditis. Their sense of frustration that this preventable disease had not yet disappeared is almost palpable.

Markowitz later worked with Leon Gordis, and the second edition of the monograph summarises some of the brilliant epidemiologic studies they made in Baltimore in the late 1960's, by which time the disease was virtually confined to a small section of the inner city. From there, happily, it "softly and silently vanished away." Perhaps not entirely silently, for a number of authors speculated on why it had gone, and whether, like tuberculosis, it might reappear. A few minioutbreaks in the late 1980s in several cities have not been followed by any upsurge.

Pediatric Cardiology and Rheumatic Fever. What role did pediatric cardiologists play in this success story? Only a few played a major part as individuals. Those with a penchant for the catheterisation laboratory, or the dramatic new therapies unfolding for heart defects, found the enigmas and protracted course of rheumatic carditis less challenging. Most of the important work was done by epidemiologists, "streptococcologists," and an interesting assorted band of pediatricians and other physicians who remained fascinated by rheumatic fever as a paradigm of a preventable and treatable disease, long after most cardiologists had shifted to congenital heart defects.

A few cardiologists, including Rachel Ash of Philadelphia [191], had early undertaken **long term follow up** studies on a cohort of patients: she found that over a 10 year period 28% of children admitted with acute rheumatic fever had died. This was perhaps the first long term follow up study of cardiac children anywhere, and as such deserves both acclaim and sympathy: acclaim for the pioneering effort to determine outcome, before the word was used, in the absence of computers, grants and effective treatment. Sympathy for the emotional toll such a discouraging mortality must have had on patients, families and staff alike. Fortunately, Rachel Ash lived long enough to see treatment begin, and the severity and incidence of the disease begin its dramatic free fall.

Several pediatric cardiologists participated in the 10-year working party study of 420 patients published in 1965 [192], an **international collaborative study** of treatment of acute rheumatic fever. This study, which helped refine the criteria of rheumatic carditis, is found today mostly as footnote to a footnote. The aim of the participants, who began the study in the early 1950s, was to establish the relative efficacy of steroids (ACTH or prednisone) compared to salicylates, which had been in use for many decades [193].

That no major difference was established between the treatment groups remained a source of interest and controversy for many years. Participating briefly in the pilot study in a very minor way, as a cardiac Fellow in Toronto, documenting murmurs, sedimentation rates, and fever levels twice weekly on a small group of patients, instilled respect if no overwhelming affection for such collaborative studies. The study established several important facts. Perhaps the most valuable was that such international collaboration was possible. There were a few areas of dissension apparent in prior reports published in earlier years of the study; possibly more existed if one were privy to the meetings of the leaders. One was the much greater frequency of the diastolic murmur of mild aortic regurgitation in Great Britain compared with the USA and Canada. The three major theories, relative deafness this side of the Atlantic, the use of stethoscopes with built in diastolic murmurs in Britain (as in Oliver Wendell Holmes poem on flies buzzing), or differing patterns of disease all had their enthusiastic proponents. A few recent Doppler echocardiographic studies have suggested that "inaudible" levels of mild aortic regurgitation are frequent in rheumatic carditis, and disappear with resolution of the active phase. The study showed a 5% mortality over the 10 year period of follow up, a fall of dramatic proportions from that recorded by Ash in the pre-therapeutic era. This collaborative study of rheumatic fever and carditis preceded by at least three decades the multi-acronymed investigations of different therapies for coronary artery disease, studies which now occupy many journals and meetings. In retrospect, it was a landmark in the study of childhood heart disease.

Many pediatric cardiologists followed their patients in rheumatic fever clinics and battled with the problems of compliance in secondary prophylaxis. It is of historic interest that several important concepts, including those of **epidemiology, patient compliance**, and **risk factors** both for disease and for non compliance were introduced into the thinking of pediatric cardiology from work in rheumatic fever [158a]. The epidemiology of rheumatic fever was well established long before that of congenital heart disease. For example, the role of overcrowding in facilitating the spread of streptococcal infection and secondary outbreaks of rheumatic fever had been documented during World War II. Ingenious research on patient compliance with drug taking regimens was undertaken by Leon Gordis, using penicillin levels in the urine, long before compliance was recognised as important in treatment of hypertension and other cardiac disorders in adults.

Changes in Rheumatic Heart Disease since 1965. As **surgical options** increased, pediatric cardiologists also had the difficult task of trying to decide when valve replacement was needed in severe chronic rheumatic heart disease. This task was made more challenging by constant changes in artificial valves, and by the lack of a really adequate tool for assessing the severity of valvar disease by non-invasive means. It is an irony of fate that mitral stenosis began to be treated successfully by valvulotomy in the 1950s, but that children in the Western world usually developed severe valvar insufficiency. If they developed mitral stenosis, it was mostly in late adolescence or early adult life.

In rheumatic fever in developing countries, by contrast, an extraordinarily rapid progression from the acute attack to severe mitral stenosis requiring early surgery or balloon valvuloplasty has been documented many times [189a]. Odell and Vosloo [194] have recently discussed the changing patterns of surgical treatment of valve disease in pediatric patients, including some of the problems presented by anti-coagulation, early calcification of bioprosthetic valves, and other problems encountered by patients, families and physicians during the pioneering years of valve surgery in children.

During the two decades since the reports of Markowitz and Kuttner, and the 10 year international study, massive external forces of social change, improved nutrition, antibiotic use, and possibly changes in streptococcal virulence [195], have been at work. In the West, rheumatic heart disease has become rare enough to present a diagnostic dilemma to the many pediatricians who have never seen a child with this once frequent problem.

Possibly the major role of pediatric cardiology as a discipline in the inexorable control of rheumatic fever has been organisational and exhortative. The Council on Cardiovascular Disease in the Young of the American Heart Association persevered in stressing the importance of primary and secondary prophylaxis of rheumatic fever to pediatricians, cardiologists, and the public; the updating of the Jones criteria for modern use [196], is but the latest of their contributions. Even after the term "rheumatic fever" disappeared from the council's title, they and their counterparts in other countries recognised that pediatric cardiology could never rest until this disease, like smallpox, passed into the oblivion of history.

MITRAL VALVE PROLAPSE

Mitral valve prolapse, quite unlike rheumatic heart disease, "appeared" on the scene of pediatric cardiology in the mid 1960s and shows no sign of disappearing [157]. Many have asked where it had been hiding: and if, as seems likely, it had always existed, how did pediatric cardiologists previously account for it? These questions, like many other tantalising ones in history, can never be satisfactorily answered. It seems likely that most children with such findings were labelled as having innocent murmurs, and the click, when heard, attributed to some unusual extracardiac variant. A few of the more unfortunate who happened to have a streptococcal infection when first seen with a murmur of mitral regurgitation, may have been thought to have rheumatic carditis; even fewer may have actually developed prolapse during the course of carditis, a sequence now well documented to occur. The Scylla and Charybdis of over- and under-labelling for rheumatic carditis was well recognised by the late 1950s, even by those who adhered rigidly to the Jones criteria.

Clicks from Capetown: Pediatric cardiologists were not alone in failing to have recognised this common problem. Cardiologists working with adults had perhaps been swifter to hear it, but did not apply the correct combination of the tools of phonocardiography and left ventricular angiography needed for elucidation.

As for pediatric cardiology, it must be remembered that in the early years of clinicophysiologic correlation and surgery, from the mid 1950s to 1970s, recognition of severe, "significant" or "organic" heart murmurs was the major focus. Much confusion was unfortunately added by widespread use of the term "flow murmur" to denote murmurs not related to structural heart defects. This term ignored the fact, well stated by Roger in the late 19th century, that all heart murmurs, including those through a ventricular septal defect, depend on active flow. (In an unavailing attempt to remove the term from use, one of us was accustomed to remind students and house staff of the complete absence of murmurs in Departments of Pathology. Changing terminology is a difficult game, as many cardiac pathologists themselves will attest). To be just, there is no evidence that pediatric cardiologists using any terminology were prescient enough to recognise prolapse.

A mid-systolic click had been recognised by Gallavardin in 1887, and thought to be extracardiac in origin. Even earlier, Sir William Osler [197] had reported "a remarkable heart murmur heard at a distance from the chest wall" in a twelve year old girl, probaly the first account of the systolic "whoop" or "honk" heard in a small minority of patients with prolapse. Although others had shown upward billowing of mitral valve leaflets in patients with late systolic murmurs [198], the term **Barlow syndrome** is still often and justly applied to mitral valve prolapse [157,199].

What tools and concepts enabled Barlow and his colleagues in Capetown to define a common syndrome which had eluded others? Probably a specific interest and skill in auscultation was their greatest weapon. Where others had been content to label this an extracardiac sound, they confirmed by phonocardiography that the click and murmur occupied a specific time in the cardiac cycle. They then localised the problem to the mitral valve using the relatively recent tool of left ventriculography. Angled views of the septum and mitral valve were less sophisticated than they became later, but even so their studies were convincing.

Dysfunction of the mitral valve apparatus was associated with a late systolic murmur preceded by a click in 15 children reported at a meeting of the American College of Cardiology in 1968 by David Schwartz and Sam Kaplan of Cincinnatti [200]. The syndrome was shortly thereafter recognised in all centers. Once echocardiography became available, many epidemiologic and family studies were undertaken. The wide spectrum of the disorder was revealed, ranging from a trivial billowing of the posterior leaflet of the mitral valve frequent in healthy children, through the severe progressive mitral regurgitation of Marfan syndrome. A number of studies sought to establish the frequency of mitral valve prolapse in mild or convalescent rheumatic carditis, the cardiomyopathy of muscular dystrophy, and other disorders. The need for meticulous echocardiograms to avoid overdiagnosis was stressed by David Sahn and others [201].

The Spectrum of MVP: In the 3 decades since Barlow defined the syndrome, the prevalence and the usual benign natural history in childhood have been well defined. The auscultatory maneuvres useful in recognising the click and murmur are now widely taught in ambulatory pediatric settings. Some question still remains if there is a subgroup of children and families in whom prolapse is complicated by panic attacks and vasomotor instability. We cannot yet predict with certainty which patients may experience embolic phenomena or which valves will progress to mitral regurgitation in adult life. There is, fortunately, increasing evidence that leaflets without either redundancy or thickening almost never degenerate.

Mitral valve prolapse entered the history of pediatric cardiology over two centuries years after Harvey wrote of the normal circulation, and one hundred and fifty years after Laennec introduced his wooden cylindrical stethoscope. It remains, a frequent and benign anomaly, in the grey hinterland between normality and disease, a land our modern tools allow us to enter but more rarely to understand.

Preventive Cardiology

Risk factors for adult heart disease were being investigated using the tools of epidemiologic and biochemical research now available. Epidemiologic investigations, including the Framingham study, were beginning to issue preliminary reports [202]. The term preventive cardiology was now part of the common language [203]. The concept that much adult cardiac disease has its origins in childhood inspired long term studies of coronary artery risk factors in children. Factors studied included serial cholesterol measurements, diet, exercise, heredity, and blood pressure. Major long term projects involving large cohorts of normal children began in Muscatine Iowa [204], Bogalusa Louisiana, and Rochester, Minnesota. The American Academy of Pediatrics and the American Heart Association collaborated on obtaining normal percentile blood pressure levels for children at various ages. Preventive cardiology became an active component of pediatric thinking and planning during the decades from the mid 1950s to 1970s.

The Pioneer Patient

Patients who underwent surgery in the first two decades of cardiopulmonary bypass were all pioneers. They were travelling in uncharted lands, just as some of their grandparents and greatgrandparents had gone across mountains and deserts in search of a new life. Some of these pioneers had come from sheltered, loving homes, brought by parents who sought health for them through the wonders of new technology. Some had fled persecution in Europe, had undergone shunt procedures when they were innovative, and now as adults faced a new operation with a hope of long term cure. The story of these pioneers has yet to be written. Many of them have become both friends and patients, and some have fine careers and families, and are reaching the slopes of aging with the courage they and their parents showed in youth. They, and those whom we lost, are part of the tapestry of pediatric cardiology.

ADDITIONAL REFERENCES AND NOTES

123. Varghese PJ, Celermajer J, Izukawa T, Haller JA Jr, Rowe RD. Cardiac catheterisation in the newborn: experience with 100 cases. Pediatrics 1969;44:24-29.

124. Rudolph AM, Heymann MA. The circulation of the fetus in utero. Methods for studying distribution of blood flow, cardiac output and organ blood flow. Circ Res 1967 21:163-184.

125. Rudolph AM, Yuan S. Response of the pulmonary vasculature to hypoxia and H+ ion concentration changes. J Clin Inv 1966;45:399-411.

126. Friedman WF, Pool PE, Jacobowitz D, Seagren SC, Braunwald E. Sympathetic innervation of the developing rabbit heart: Biochemical and histochemical comparisons of fetal, neonatal and adult rabbit myocardium. Circulation Research 1968;23:25-32.

127. Smith DW Recognizable patterns of human malformation: genetic embryologic and clinical aspects. Philadelphia: Saunders, 1970.

127a Smith DW, Jones KL. Smith's recognisable patterns of human malformations. 4th ed. Philadelphia Saunders 1988.

128. Rosenquist GC, De Haan RL. Migration of precardiac cells in the chick embryo: A radioautographic study. Carnegie Contributions Embryology 1966; 38:111-115.

129. Pexieder T. Cell death in the morphogenesis and teratogenesis of the heart. Adv Anat Embryol Cell Biol 1975;51:1-100.

130. Rychter Z. Experimental morphology of the aortic arches and the heart loop in chick embryos. Adv Morphogen 1962;2:333-371.

131. Clark EB, Hu N. Developmental hemodynamic changes in the chick embryo stages 18 to 27. Circ Res 1983;51:810-815.

132. Wilson JG, Warkany J. Aortic arch and cardiovascular anomalies in the offspring of vitamin A deficient rats. Pediatrics 1948;1:462-468.

133. Fox MH, Goss CM. Experimentally produced malformations of the heart and great vessels in rat fetuses. Anat Rec 1957;129:309-331.

134. Kalter H, Warkany J. Experimental production of congenital malformations in mammals by metabolic procedures. Physiol Rev 1959;39:69-115.

135. Swan C, Tostevin AL, Moore B, Mayo H, Barham Black GH. Congenital defects in infants following infectious diseases during pregnancy, with special reference to relationship between German measles and cataract, deaf mutism, heart disease and microcephaly, and to period of pregnacy in which occurrence of rubella is followed by congenital abnormalities. Med J Austr 1943;2:201-210.

136. Rowe RD. Maternal rubella and pulmonary artery stenosis. Report of eleven cases. Pediatrics 1963;32:180-185.

137. Lenz W, Knapp K. Fetal malformations due to thalidomide. German Med Monthly 1962;7:253-258.

138. Taussig HB. A study of the German outbreak of phocomelia—The Thalidomide Syndrome. JAMA 1962; 180:1106-1114.

139. Fraser FC, Lenz W, Warkany J, Kelsey FO, Heshka T, Stephens TD, Brent RL, Holmes LB. Thalidomide Symposium. Teratology 1988;38:201-241.

140. Lipson AH. Thalidomide retrospective: What did the clinical teratologist learn? Teratology 1992;46:411-413.

141. Lammer EJ, Chen DT, Hoar RM, et al. Retinoic acid embryopathy. New Eng J Med 1985;313:837-841.

142. Williams JCP, Barratt-Boyes BG, Lowe JB. Supravalvar aortic stenosis. Circulation 1961; 24:1311-1318.

143. Black JA, Bonham Carter RE. Association between aortic stenosis, peripheral pulmonary stenosis, mental retardation, and similar facial appearance. Lancet 1963;2:745-748.

144. Beuren AJ, Schulze C, Eberle P, Harmanz D, Apitz A. The syndrome of supravalvar aortic stenosis, peripheral pulmonary stenosis, mental retardation, and similar facial appearance. Am J Cardiol 1964;13:471-483.

145. Ewart AK, Morris CA, Atkinson D, et al. Hemizygosity at the elastin locus in a developmental disorder, Williams syndrome. Nature Genet 1993;5:11-16.

146. Mitchell SC, Sellman AH, Westphal MC, Park J. Etiologic correlates in a study of congenital heart disease in 56,109 live births. Am J Cardiol 1971;23:653-657.

147. Polani PE, Campbell M. An aetiologic study of congenital heart disease. Ann Hum Genet 1955;19:209-230.

148. Lamy M, De Grouchy J, Schweisguth O. Genetic and non-genetic factors in the etiology of congenital heart disease: A study of 1188 cases. Am J Hum Genet 1957;9:17-41.

149. Patterson DF, Detweiler DK. Hereditary transmission of patent ductus arteriosus in the dog. Am Heart J 1967;74:289-290.

150. Rowe RD, Uchida IA. Cardiac malformation in mongolism: a prospective study of 184 mongoloid children. Am J Med 1961;31:726-735.

151. Lejeune J, Gauthier M, Turpin R. Etude des chromosomes somatiques de neuf enfants mongoliens. Comptes Rend Acad Science Paris 1959; 248:1721-1722.

152. Kibrick S, Benirschke K. Acute aseptic myocarditis and meningoencephalitis in the newborn child infected with Cocksackie virus group B type 3. New Eng J Med 1956;255:883-889.

153. Goodwin JF, Hollman A, Cleland WP, Teare RD. Obstructive cardiomyopathy simulating aortic stenosis. Brit Heart J 1960;22:403-414.

154. Johnson DH, Rosenthal A, Nadas AS. A forty-year review of bacterial endocarditis in infancy and childhood. Circulation 1975;51:581-588.

155. Simcha A, Bonham Carter RE. Paroxysmal atrial tachycardia in infants and children. Lancet 1971;1: 832-834.

156. Kawasaki T. Acute febrile mucocutaneous syndrome with lymphoid involvement with specific desquamation of the fingers and toes in infants and children: Clinical observation in 50 cases. Japan J Allergy 1967;16:178-222.

157. Barlow JB, Pocock WA, Marchand P, Denny M. The significance of the late systolic murmur. Am Heart J 1963;66:443-452.

158. Markowitz M, Kuttner AG. Rheumatic Fever. Philadelphia: WB Saunders, 1965.

158a. 2nd edition Markowitz M, Gordis L ibid 1972.

159. Swan H, Zeavin I, Blount SG, Virtue RW. Surgery by direct vision in the open heart during hypothermia. JAMA 1953; 153:1081-1085.

160. Bigelow WG. Cold Hearts: The story of hypothermia and the pacemaker in heart surgery. Toronto: McClelland and Stewart, 1984.

161. Lillehei CW, Cohen M, Warden HE, Varco RL. The direct vision intracardiac correction of congenital anomalies by controlled cross circulation. Results in thirty two patients with ventricular septal defects, tetralogy of Fallot, and atrioventricular communis defects. Surg 1955;38:11-29.

162. Gibbon JH Jr. Application of a mechanical heart and lung apparatus to cardiac surgery. Minnesota Med 1954;37:171-185.

163. Hewitt RL, Creech O Jr. History of the pump oxygenator. Arch Surg 1966;93:680-696.

164. Kirklin JW, DuShane JW, Patrick RT, Donald DE, Hetzel PS, Harshbarger HG, Wood EH. Intracardiac surgery with the aid of a mechanical pump-oxygenator system (Gibbon type): Report of eight cases. Proc Staff Meetings Mayo Clin 1955;30:201-206.

165. Lev M. The architecture of the conduction system in congenital heart disease. I. Common atrioventricular orifice. Arch Path 1958;65:174-191.

166. Hutchins GM. Coarctation of the aorta as a branch-point of the ductus arteriosus. Am J Path 1971;63:203-209.

167. Roberts WC. Anatomically isolated aortic valvular disease: The case against its being of rheumatic etiology. Am J Med 1970;49:151-159.

168. Campbell M, Neill C, Suzman S. The prognosis in atrial septal defect. Brit Med J 1957;1:1375-1383.

169. Watson H. Natural history of Ebstein's anomaly of the tricuspid valve in children and adolescents: An international cooperative study of 505 cases. Brit Heart J 1974;36: 417-427.

170. Evans JR, Rowe RD, Keith JD. Spontaneous closure of ventricular septal defects. Circulation 1960;22: 1044-1054.

171. Nadas AS, Ellison RC, Weidman WH editors. Report from the Joint Study of the Natural History of Congenital Heart Defects: Pulmonary stenosis, aortic stenosis, ventricular septal defect: Clinical course and indirect assessment. Circulation 1977;56 (suppl):1-87.

172. Morriss JH, McNamara DG. Residua, sequelae, and complications of surgery for congenital heart disease. In: Postoperative congenital heart disease. Rosenthal A, Sonnenblick EH, Lesch M editors. New York, Grune and Stratton 1975:3-27.

172a. Keane JF, Williams R, Treves S, Rosenthal A. Assessment of the postoperative patient by noninvasive techniques. ibid 1975:81-98.

173. Senning A. Surgical correction for transposition of the great vessels. Surg 1959;45: 966-972.

174. Mustard WT. Successful two-stage correction of transposition of the great vessels. Surg 1964;55:469-472.

175. Rashkind WJ, Miller WW. Creation of an atrial septal defect without thoracotomy: A palliative approach to complete transposition of the great arteries. JAMA 1966;196:991-992.

176. McNamara DG. Twenty-five years of progress in the medical treatment of pediatric and congenital heart disease. J Am Coll Cardiol 1983;1:264-273.

177. Cheng TO. Percutaneous balloon valvuloplasty Cheng TO editor New York Igaku-Shoin 1992.

177a. Anderson, R.H., Becker A. E., Anatomy and Pathology of Valvular Stenosis. In: Cheng ibid p. 12-39

178. Ross DN, Somerville J. Correction of pulmonary atresia with a homograft aortic valve. Lancet 1966;2:1446-1447.

179. Rastelli GC, Wallace RB, Ongley PA. Complete repair of transposition of the great arteries with pulmonary stenosis. A review and report of a case using a new surgical technique. Circulation 1969;39:83-95.

180. Lowe JE, German LD. Cardiac pacemakers and cardiac conduction system abnormalities. In: Surgery of the Chest. Sabiston DC, Spencer FC, editors. 5th ed. Philadelphia, WB Saunders, 1990:1597-1634.

181. Gillette PC, Garson A Jr. Pediatric arrhythmias: electrophysiology and pacing. Philadelphia, WB Saunders 1990.

182. Rastelli GC, Ongley PA, Kirklin JW, McGoon DC. Surgical repair of the complete form of persistent common atrioventricular canal. J Thorac Cardiovasc Surg 1968;55:299-308.

183. Fontan F, Baudet E. Surgical repair of tricuspid atresia. Thorax 1971; 26:240-248.

184. Gerard R, Lasry F, Seichter J, Malfroy P, Jouve A. Les criteres electocardiographiques de surcharge ventriculaire droite chez l'enfant. I. Les surcharges systoliques. Arch Mal Coeur Vaiss 1969;62:1049-1071.

185. Graham TP, Jarmakani JM, Atwood GF, Canent RV. Right ventricular volume determinations in children. Normal values and observations with volume and pressure overload. Circulation 1973;47:144-153.

186. Brandt PWT, Clarkson PM, Neutze JM, Barratt-Boyes BG. Left ventricular cineangiography in endocardial cushion defect (persistent common atrioventricular canal). Austr J Radiol 1972;16:367-376.

187. Bargeron LM, Elliott LP, Soto B, Bream PR, Currey GC. Axial angiography in congenital heart disease. Section I. Concept, technical and anatomical considerations. Circulation 1977;56:1075-1083.

188. Fyler DC, Buckley LP, Hellenbrand WE, Cohn HE. Report of the New England Regional Infant Cardiac Program. Pediatrics 1980;65 (suppl):375-461.

189. Lewis BS, Gotsman MS. Natural history of rheumatic heart disease in childhood. In: Rheumatic valvular disease in children. Borman JB, Gotsman MS editors Berlin Springer Verlag 1980: 59-71.

189a. Paul ATS Closed mitral commisurotomy in children. ibid 1980:126-148.

190. Thomas CB, France R. A preliminary report of the prophylactic use of sulfanilamide in patients susceptible to rheumatic fever. Bull Johns Hopkins Hosp 1939;64:67-69.

191. Ash R. The first 10 years of rheumatic infection in childhood. Am Heart J 1948;36: 89-93.

192. Ten-year report by the Rheumatic Fever Working Party. The natural history of rheumatic fever and rheumatic heart disease. Circulation 1965;32:457-476.

193. Coburn AF, Salicylate therapy in rheumatic fever. A rational technique. Bull Johns Hopkins Hosp 1943; 73:435-464.

194. Odell JA, Vosloo SM. Valvular surgery in children. In: Valvular heart disease. Zaibag MA, Duran CMG editors New York Marcel Dekker 1994:635-656.

195. Ayoub EM, Barret DJ, Maclaren NK, Kricher P. Association of class II human histocompatibility leucocyte antigens with rheumatic fever. J Clin Inv 1986;77:2019-2026.

196. Dajani AS, Bisno AL, Kyung JC et al. Prevention of rheumatic fever. A statement for health professionals by the committe on rheumatic fever, endocarditis and Kawasaki disease of the Council on Cardiovascular Disease in the Young. Circulation 1988;78:1082-1086.

197. Osler W. On a remarkable heart murmur heard at a distance from the chest wall Can Med Surg J 1879-1880; 8:518-519.

198. Jeresaty RM. Mitral valve prolapse. New York: Raven Press, 1979.

199. Barlow JB, Bosman CK, Pocock WA et al Late systolic murmurs and non- ejection (mid-late) systolic clicks: an analysis of 90 patients Br Heart J 1968;30:203-218.

200. Schwartz DC, Daoud G, Kaplan S. Dysfunction of the mitral apparatus in children. Am J Cardiol (abst) 1968;21:114.

201. Sahn DJ, Wood J, Allen HD, et al. Echocardiographic spectrum of mitral valve motion in children with and without mitral valve prolapse: the nature of false postive diagnosis Am J Cardiol 1977;39:422-431.

202. Truett J, Cornfield J, Kannel W. A multivariate analysis of the risk of coronary heart disease in Framingham. J Chron Dis 1967.20:511-524.

203. White PD. The tardy growth of preventive cardiology. Am J Cardiol 1972; 29:886-888.

204. Lauer RM, Connor WE, Leaverton PE, Reiter MA, Clarke WR. Coronary heart disease risk factors in school children-The Muscatine study. J Pediatr. 1975;86:697-702.

CHAPTER 6

Infant Era mid 1970s to 1990

- Modern Times: Concepts of neonatal cardiology
- Tools: pharmacologic manipulation of ductus
  Doppler echocardiography
- Infant heart surgery
- Pulmonary valvuloplasty, invasive cardiology
- Kawasaki disease: cardiomyopathy: arrhythmia
- Two young women with palpitations

"In the Renaissance, knowledge of the past was not believed to be of primary significance–neither for explaining the structure of the social world nor for understanding and judging human action. History was not highly esteemed ... One of the most proudly held assumptions of the men of the Renaissance was that they lived in a time different from the past, in a new and better world ... Emphasis on the value of novelty, however, casts a shadow over what is old. A modern psychologist has said, 'New ideas, new movements, new countries, all act at first as if they were superseding history'"

—Gilbert F. The Renaissance interest in history. In: Art, Science and History in the Renaissance. Singleton CS editor. Baltimore Johns Hopkins Press 1967:373-374; quoting Erikson EH, Insight and Responsibility. New York 1964:211.

C: INFANT CARDIOLOGY ERA

Introduction

Anyone reading this chapter who is less than 45 years old will never have worked in pediatric cardiology before the "infant era," starting in the mid 1970's. We have now reached modern times, and being so close to the era makes it more difficult to assess the value of each individual contribution. This era is the topic of an increasing number of excellent textbooks on pediatric cardiology, childhood heart surgery, pediatric arrhythmias and Doppler echocardiography. Several texts deal solely with fetal and neonatal heart disease and with infant heart surgery. Those wishing to learn more of modern times in childhood heart disease certainly have no dearth of reading material. In this chapter the references are chiefly to papers and books which allow for further study of current knowledge. Future generations will have to decide if the infant era marked a "Renaissance" period for pediatric cardiology.

During the infant era, as pediatric cardiology moved into modern times, several new concepts and tools emerged which effected a radical change in thinking, management and patient outcome. These changes resulted from new concepts of neonatal and infant cardiology, including the growth of intracardiac repair in infancy; pharmacologic manipulation of the ductus; and the advent of echocardiography. Pulmonary valuloplasty ushered in the rise of invasive cardiology. At the same time, interest was growing in fetal cardiology and in the adult with congenital heart disease. Arrhythmias, cardiomyopathies and Kawasaki syndrome came under intensive study. Thus, though this was the infant era, the vision of the 4 domains of pediatric cardiology was expanding rapidly.

NEONATAL AND INFANT CARDIOLOGY

It was recognised by the 1960's that the major mortality from childhood heart disease was in infancy. Rowe and Mehrizi [205] in their 1968 monograph defined neonatal cardiology as an entity. Fyler et al [188], had shown on a regional basis the clinical spectrum of infants under one year of age requiring hospitalisation and cardiac catheterisation between 1968 and 1974. Thus the problems of infant heart disease were conceptualised, but further treatment advances depended on both research and technical changes.

The Forgotten Infant. Future historians will probably ask: why did it take so long to recognise that infancy was the crucial time of life for someone born with a heart defect? From the beginnings of cardiac history to the middle of the twentieth century is a long time. This may well be a topic for future research by medical historians, and only a few speculations can be offered here. Certainly severe heart defects had been recognised in infants at least since the 18th century. It seems likely that such defects made a very small impact on infant mortality when neonatal sepsis, gastroenteritis and respiratory illness were the great killers.

Neonatal cyanosis, in particular, would have been attributed to lung disease, and autopsy or publication of abnormal cardiac findings in a young infant must have required a special intensity from a pediatrician early in the 20th century. Also, at least until the publication of Maude Abbott's Atlas in 1936, terminology and classification was complicated and contentious enough to deter many from writing on the subject.

Even when therapy became available in the 1940's, parents at first had to travel far for care for the child. The number of centers was very limited. Although the importance of transposition as a cause of death was known by the 1940's, these infants were usually too acutely sick to travel. Thus in the early years of surgery older infants and children and even adults were the ones who came for care.

Once pediatric cardiology and cardiac surgery became more widespread, the new centers found their own patient population differed from that observed at most places of regional referral. The children tended to be younger and sicker, and to have more extracardiac malformations. The Hospital for Sick Children in Toronto occupied a special position, drawing attention to heart disease in infancy earlier than others. John Keith and his colleagues established a Heart Registry in Toronto, and were among the first to gather diagnostic and outcome data on a regional basis [206]. Remaining the only referral center for the whole Province of Ontario, they were among the earliest to recognise the high mortality in infants, and the distribution of cardiac malformations involved.

Changes in Infant Cardiology in the Infant Era. The approximately 15 years from the mid 1970's to 1990 witnessed profound changes in pediatric cardiology. Successful intracardiac repair in infancy became a reality. Other major advances occurred in neonatal and perioperative care, especially in the advent of prostaglandin therapy. Echocardiography, as it became increasingly sophisticated and included Doppler and color Doppler technology, allowed for rapid non invasive diagnosis in infancy, improving the speed of medical management and the accuracy of postoperative assessment.

OTHER CHANGES IN PEDIATRIC CARDIOLOGY

The introduction of pulmonary valvuloplasty by Jean Kan and her colleagues in 1982 [207] was followed by the rise of invasive cardiology. Kawasaki syndrome was recognised world wide during this era, and became the subject of international collaborative study. Although arrhythmias and cardiomyopathy had always existed, they now became major areas of investigation for pediatric cardiologists. New collaborative ventures with geneticists and epidemiologists brought realisation that cardiac syndromes were both more widespread and significant than once thought. Cardiac nurse specialists assumed a major role in patient care and follow up in all centers, and helped improve communication with families in what was now a fast moving and constantly changing specialty.

Cardiac transplantation, and the use of extracorporeal membrane oxygenators for critically ill infants and children, were beneficial for a few individuals, and stimulated further research on the myocardium and cardiopulmonary interactions.

During this same era, many of the patients treated at the dawn of therapy were reaching adult life and even middle age. Questions of who should care for them, their employability, quality of life, pregnancy and genetic risks came under active discussion in papers and seminars. Fortunately, most of the pioneer patients handled these questions themselves with great sang-froid, sometimes with a little help from their friends, the pediatric cardiologists. But for a few with pulmonary vascular obstructive disease or complex defects, adult life was hazardous and at times distressing. Jane Somerville of London was one of the very few cardiologists who constantly reminded her colleagues of the needs of those for whom the modern age of therapy had not been a golden one.

Although most pediatric cardiologists spent their time, as in the past, chiefly in patient care, their specialty was changing around them even faster than was academic medicine as a whole. Their writings during this era overwhelmingly dealt with the application of new diagnostic tools. As was true of the men of the Renaissance described in the chapter heading, "history was not highly esteemed."

The Normal Heart

The hemodynamics of the normal heart was a subject now well understood, and little was added during this period from cardiac catheterisation techniques. The physiology of the fetal, neonatal and adult heart was now thought of as a continuum, and much research was devoted to exploring changes with maturation [208].

The advent of echocardiography allowed for new correlations between anatomy and physiology in a wider range of ages than possible earlier. Accurate reproducible measurements made of ventricular wall thickness, aortic root size, and atrial and ventricular cavity dimensions, led to a more dynamic concept of the changes in the heart with growth.

These new echocardiographic studies were later useful in documenting some of the progressive changes of disease, for example the steadily increasing dilatation of the aortic root with age in Marfan syndrome, or the changes in left ventricular wall thickness with adolescent hypertension.

Other methods of imaging the heart played a lesser role in pediatrics than in evaluating the adult heart. Magnetic resonance imaging was useful in allowing for differentiation of normal from abnormal myocardium, and in the imaging of heterotaxies.

The myocardium could now be studied by cardiac biopsy [209], and new microscopic techniques were used to differentiate myocarditis or metabolic derangements from normal heart muscle. Biochemical reactions in the normal heart and in heart failure were evaluated.

In pediatric cardiology, the impact of echocardiography was overwhelming. With the fluoroscope, one could see the heart, in the words of Saint Paul, "through a glass, darkly." Fascinating though it is as a tool of diagnosis, the greatest gift of the echocardiogram lies in its visualisation of the normal infant heart, the fragile toughness of the mitral valve, the elegance of the stability of structure, yet the capacity to change and grow. It is a wonderful gift to modern times.

The Developing Heart

A number of laboratories around the world were now studying the embryonic heart, using experimental alterations in embryonic flows and pressures, electron microscopy, teratology and animal models. In 1978 Atsuyoshi Takao began a series of

International Symposia on cardiac development in Tokyo. The reports of the first three of these symposia entitled "Etiology and morphogenesis," "Causes and processes" and "Developmental cardiology: Morphogenesis and function" chart the extraordinary explosion of new knowledge during the 15 years of the infant era [210].

The demonstration by Kirby et al in 1983 [211] of the role of neural crest cells in aortopulmonary septation provided a major stimulus to new clinical and genetic concepts of conotruncal syndromes. The role of **neural crest cells** was studied experimentally [210], and the recognition of retinoic acid embryopathy by Lammer and associates in 1985 [141] increased clinical awareness of the association of conotruncal and branchial arch defects.

In 1986 Clark proposed the concept of **developmental mechanisms** [212], which proved liberating as a new approach to grouping of defects in epidemiologic and family studies.

Research into possible genetic mechanisms of cardiac defects, which earlier had mainly involved clinical family studies [213,214], could now be approached with the tools of microbiology [215,216]. This research technique has led to understanding of the specific defect underlying Marfan syndrome, and also allows for exclusion of the diagnosis in children and adults who share some features of the phenotype. Precision of diagnosis at the level of molecular biology will prove an extremely valuable tool in the previously inexact field of genetic counselling.

Human research designed to include both genetic and environmental prenatal risk factors presents formidable challenges. These challenges began to be systematically addressed with the start of the Baltimore Washington Infant Study in 1981 [217]. Charlotte Ferencz's report on her monumental 10 year study is an international resource, whose contents will be studied for decades to come.
Her introductory chapter, describing the influences which led her into this research endeavor, is in itself part of the history of pediatric cardiology. Instead of quoting from this chapter, we recommend that it be read.

Heart Disease and Defects in Infancy

Surgical and medical advances were rapid and sweeping during the period beginning in the mid 1970's, which we have called the infant era. Others will undoubtedly label it the age of ultrasound, and that is true, but limiting. Ultrasound is not only valuable in infants, but it made the infant era possible.

In preparation for writing this chapter we compared the reports of two medical meetings, four years apart. The first was held in 1972 at Key Biscayne Florida; the meeting was described by Sidney Blumenthal in his foreword [218] as one called to review the current status and training needs of the discipline of pediatric cardiology. Several important papers were presented, including William Rashkind's discussion of historic aspects of congenital heart disease [24]. At this gathering of prominent pediatric cardiologists there was no mention of echocardiography, although some echocardiograms had already been reported in children [219]. At the second meeting, an international symposium in 1976, held in honor of Helen Taussig [220], two papers show reproductions of M-mode echocardiograms, primitive by standards of today, yet illustrative of how this new tool would prove useful in noninvasive documentation of left atrial enlargement and in septal hypertrophy. In discussion of a case report of a premature infant dying with a patent ductus arteriosus, mention is made of a new collaborative study of indomethacin. The reports of these two meetings provide evidence that a new era began in the mid 1970's, and that infants were profoundly affected.

In McNamara's analysis of twenty-five years of progress in the medical treatment of pediatric and congenital heart disease [176], he includes echocardiography, pharmacologic manipulation of the ductus, and advances in the technology of catheterisation as among the most important. Cardiac catheterisation in infants and children was improved by use of miniaturised equipment, control of body temperature, the introduction of the image intensifier and biplane cineangiography, and better angiographic views. New methods of sedation and the use of percutaneous techniques all resulted in safer studies with a higher yield of useful information, particularly in small infants.

Pharmacologic Manipulation of the Ductus was a critically important advance of the infant era. The concept of such manipulation [221] built on much prior work on the responsiveness of ductal musculature to oxygen, prostaglandins and prostaglandin inhibitors. Coccean̈i and Olley showed in 1973 that the ductus could be dilated by **prostaglandin E_1** in fetal lambs. Others confirmed their experiments, and Peter Olley and his colleagues in 1976 [222] went on to describe the concept of 'duct dependent' lesions and their role in neonatal mortality. As with many other concepts, the idea that ductal flow was important had been voiced before, but Olley not only articulated his concept with unrivalled clarity, but made the concept of practical use in infancy by a combination of elegant experimental and clinical work. He wrote:

> *"Congenital heart defects which include pulmonary atresia, critical pulmonary stenosis or a severely hypoplastic right ventricle as part of the malformation are frequently almost entirely dependent on persistence of the ductus arteriosus for the maintenance of pulmonary blood flow. Likewise interruption of the aortic arch requires ductus patency for blood flow to the lower half of the body."*

Now that prostaglandins are in such widespread use in cyanotic newborn infants, it is fortunately hard to remember the vicious downhill spiral seen in some infants in the 1960's, as progressive acidemia followed spontaneous ductal closure. Early referral and safe transportation to regional cardiac centers now became the norm of infant care.

Effecting ductal closure by the use of indomethacin, a prostaglandin inhibitor, was another valuable advance for certain infants, though it had a less revolutionary impact on pediatric cardiology. Many studies had shown that a persistent ductus was often present in premature infants, but it was not till the late 1960's that the maligant combination of low birth weight, respiratory distress, and a large, sometimes clinically "silent" patent ductus began to be recognised. Some successful surgical ligations were reported, but accurate assessment of ductal shunt size was difficult prior to echocardiography, and there was much incentive to find if the duct could be medically closed. Friedman [223] was among the pioneers in the use of indomethacin, and a large multicenter trial soon followed. The almost simultaneous introduction of echocardiogaphy was helpful, making it possible to follow the course of the duct; at first, only the relatively crude M-mode analysis of the left atrial to aortic root ratio was used, but later, with Doppler echocardiography, the duct itself could be seen and the shunt visualised.

Unlike some other fields of endeavor, with pharmacologic manipulation of the ductus the concept and production of the requisite medications, the tools of therapy, evolved within a relatively short time span: both tools and concept are now used daily in critically ill neonates around the world.

INTRACARDIAC REPAIR IN INFANCY

Cardiac surgeons had successfully performed intracardiac repairs in infancy in the 1950's to 1970's. For the most part, however, these were isolated triumphs. Sir Brian Barratt-Boyes of Auckland, New Zealand [224], and Aldo Castaneda of Boston [225] were leaders in further progress, including the use of miniaturised equipment and hypothermic cardiac arrest.

As had happened after the Blalock Taussig shunt, successful techniques were rapidly adopted by other centers [226], and new procedures were introduced [227,228]. Spurred by Kirklin and his colleagues in Alabama, the new tool of rigorous statistical analysis began to be applied to outcome studies.

Complete transposition was now being treated worldwide by the Mustard or Senning type of intraatrial repair. The longer follow up continued, the more it became apparent that the patients, despite normal oxygenation and an almost normal life style, faced progressive atrial arrhyhthmias and right ventricular dysfunction. In 1976 Jatene of Sao Paulo, Brazil [229] succesfully transformed the concept of arterial switch for transposition into a dramatic and life saving reality, one which rapidly came into international use. An unprecedented collaborative study was undertaken [230], and the value of the new procedure was quickly established [231,232].

Complete transposition is often cited as the paradigm of progress in pediatric cardiology [233]. Infants born with this defect, once almost uniformly fatal in the first month of life only eleven years earlier, could now have immediate neonatal diagnosis by echocardiography, transport to a regional center on prostaglandins, and an arterial switch in the first few days of life, often without the need for cardiac catheterisation. They were never exposed to the hazards of profound hypoxia, acidosis, and multiple interventions faced by their predecessors. If postoperative problems arose, such as stenosis at the anastomotic site in the aorta or pulmonary artery, these could be detected by echocardiography and mostly treated by balloon catheter dilatation without further surgery. This progress had indeed been remarkable, possibly unprecedented in medical history.

Other cardiac defects shared in these advances to varying degrees. Anyone who had once followed an infant with total anomalous pulmonary venous return through the inexorable downhill course characterised by heart failure and profound growth retardation, recognised the surgeon's ability to perform repair in the neonate as a dramatic and gratifying advance. An infant with a large ventricular septal defect no longer needed repeated admissions for management of congestive heart failure. Those days were over. As ventriculotomies were increasingly avoided in favor of an atrial approach to repair of ventricular defects, many of the postoperative problems of myocardial dysfunction ceased.

The best management of tetralogy of Fallot was debated for some years, and some advocated the prophylactic use of propranalol or shunt procedures in infancy, and repair at an optimal size or weight. With the "movement of cardiac surgery to the very young," so brilliantly outlined by John Kirklin in 1989 [234], a consensus was gradually reached that repair in early infancy avoided the many difficulties, including progression of right ventricular hypertrophy. New postoperative strategies greatly improved the outcome for early repair of complete atrioventricular septal defects. Because of the rapid development of pulmonary vascular obstructive disease [235], infants with Down syndrome needed open repair of such defects before six months of age.

The widening gulf. As more and more complex defects became approachable, the kaleidoscope of therapy shifted yet again. If complete transposition, or infradiaphragmatic anomalous pulmonary venous return, were the paradigms, being defects treatable in the neonatal period with a strong possibility of cure after one brief hospitalisation, who were the exceptions? Did every child born with a heart defect have a future so bright and free of long term hazards. There has been great difficulty in defining the answer to this question in precise terms. It may be one of the difficulties of pediatric cardiology at the beginning of the 1990's that this question has rarely been asked. Pediatricians and families, and sometimes cardiologists and surgeons, have faced with reluctance the possibility that multiple interventions are still needed for some cardiac defects, and that heart surgery cannot result in a normal child in the presence of a syndrome or multiple extracardiac anomalies.

The gulf has widened between the course of infants born with two adequate ventricles and no extracardiac anomalies, for whom heart surgery, as in complete transposition, could be curative; and those with a hypoplastic ventricle [236], or severe extracardiac anomalies [237], who often needed multiple interventions, and whose extracardiac problems remained even after cardiac correction.

ECHOCARDIOGRAPHY

The use of ultrasound waves in submarine detection during World War II had alerted scientists to their potential value. However, the development of appropriate transducers, imaging systems and methods of data retrieval took many years and significant changes in concepts and technology. From the point of view of the sick infant with heart disease, echocardiography could not have been introduced at a better time. Sydney Blumenthal, in his brief overview of pediatric cardiology in 1972 [218], commented:

> *Pediatric cardiology has been emerging from a period of rapid growth in which tremendous progress was made in a short span of years. Descriptive analyses of new clinical syndromes and documentation of their hemodynamic pathophysiology have been almost exhausted . . ."*

He was probably referring to "syndromes" with multiple cardiac anomalies, such as the scimitar or Shone syndrome, for in fact the understanding of the association of cardiac and extracardiac anomalies was only beginning. But it was true that little remained to be learnt of the hemodynamics of heart defects in the catheterisation laboratory. A new way of seeing the heart was needed.

Anyone who has grown up in the era of ultrasound will find it difficult to imagine life without it. The clinical profiles that had led to diagnosis in the past were constructed like a series of building blocks, or patches in a quilt, so that several observations joined to make a structural diagnosis. For example, to return to Maude Abbott's Atlas, coarctation of the aorta in the adult was a diagnosis built on clinical observation of upper extremity hypertension, palpation of dilated pulsating intercostal arteries, rib notching on chest radiograph, and left ventricular hypertrophy on the electrocardiogram: all findings which were helpful in adults, but obscure or absent in infancy. The findings in adults were consequences or sequelae of prolonged physiologic derangement acting over many years. With the advent of aortography, the coarctation itself could be visualised, but the dynamic nature of the defect was never fully appreciated until Doppler echocardiography. Most writing on echocardiography stresses, correctly, its value in diagnosis. But its drama lies in the ability to see the chambers and vessels of the beating heart as no generation has ever seen them before. Anatomy and physiology are together in the image.

An Evolving Technique: Clinical echocardiography began rather modestly, and probably only those who worked actively with the physicists and engineers involved had any concept of how sophisticated a tool it would soon become. The principles and techniques underlying its use have been well described in many papers and textbooks. The direct imaging of the heart by ultrasound was a remarkable contribution to this infant era. Even in the early years the value of the technique in assessing complex anomalies, such as atrioventricular septal defect, was appreciated [238].

The rapid advance from M-mode to two dimensional sections [239] provided the cardiologist with a unique window on the beating heart. Pulsed and continuous wave doppler measured blood velocity and provided indirect measurement of intracardiac pressure differences. As color Doppler technology became available, even tiny left to right shunts could be visualised. These new tools not only revolutionised the practice of pediatric cardiology, but brought physiologic concepts into daily use in the ambulatory setting.

Intracardiac anatomy, cardiac physiology and myocardial function could now be assessed at all ages, freed from the constraints and ordeals of the cardiac catheterisation laboratory. Rebecca Snider, one of the leaders in the technique [240], has emphasised the recent move of echocardiography from pure "qualitative description to quantitative assessment," whether of myocardial mass, shunt size, or ventricular function. Transesophageal echocardiography provided unequalled access to the atrial septum and atrioventricular valves, and proved particularly valuable intra-operatively and in the intensive care setting.

As ultrasound technology improved, the human fetal heart, long hidden deep within the uterus, became accessible. Fetal echocardiography [241,242] stimulated the need to understand cardiac development; an annual series of international symposia on the techniques and implications of the technique began in 1977. Fetal echocardiography provided a simultaneous picture of the anatomy and physiology of the growing heart inside the mother. It also, in a few cases, provided new and difficult areas of prenatal counselling when an intracardiac defect was discovered. These difficulties were counteracted by the many opportunities for reassurance that a structurally normal heart was present despite some risk factor such as maternal diabetes.

The use of Doppler echocardiography (Fig 11) has proved invaluable in assessing pressure gradients across stenotic valves, or between the two ventricles, and has markedly decreased the need for invasive hemodynamic studies to make such determinations.

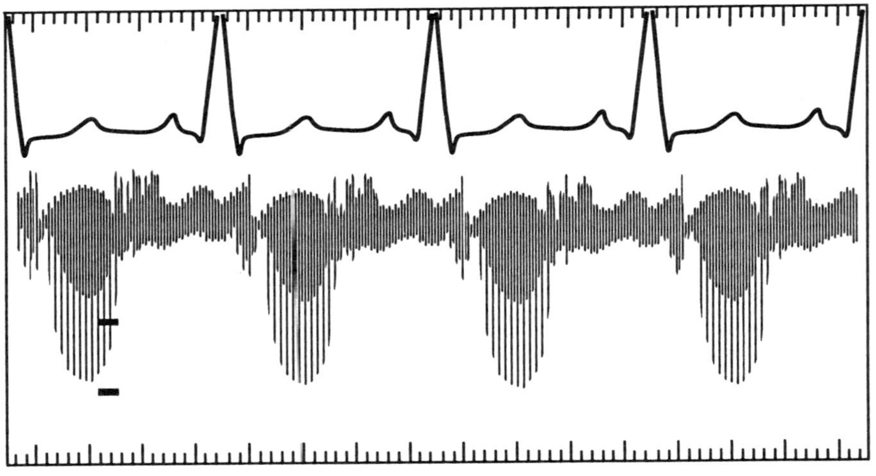

Figure 11. Diagram simulating how Doppler echocardiography can be used in non invasive assessment of intracardiac pressure gradients.

PULMONARY VALVULOPLASTY

Dilatation of a stenotic pulmonary valve with a balloon catheter is a procedure of value at all ages, not confined to infancy. It can, however, provide dramatic relief in the neonatal period to the rare infant born with critically severe pulmonary valve stenosis.

The procedure was introduced in 1982 by Jean Kan and her colleagues of Johns Hopkins in Baltimore. Her coauthors included Timothy Gardner of cardiovascular surgery and Robert White and Sally Mitchell of cardiovascular radiology [207]. The authorship of the paper symbolises the team approach of modern pediatric cardiology. The radiologists had access to the new instruments being developed since coronary angioplasty had become possible, and surgical support and expertise was invaluable in the pioneering days. Every team needs a leader, and Jean Kan's combination of brilliance and patience in the catheterisation laboratory made her the director of this project, and a continuing expert in the field.

In some of her talks on the history of balloon valvuloplasty she starts with a picture of Rambo, a large and amiable, if unprepossessing, English bulldog, who had allowed his congenitally stenotic pulmonary valve to be dilated prior to any human trial. Rambo, like the many thousands of humans who have by now succeeded him, did well. The diagram [below] (Fig 12), illustrates the changing appearance of the catheter before and after valve dilatation.

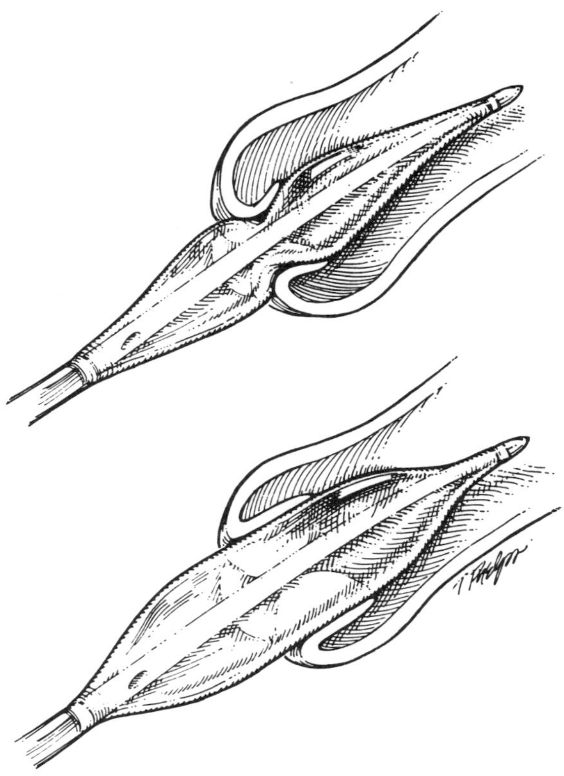

Figure 12 Balloon catheter used in pulmonary valvulopasty. After dilatation of the valve, the "waisting" of the balloon at the level of the valve is no longer seen. (redrawn, with permission, from Kan et al 1982 [207].

The value of the new technique was rapidly confirmed in many other centers, and following a large multicenter trial became the accepted method of treatment. Sixteen years had passed since Rashkind had used a balloon catheter to enlarge the atrial septal defect in transposition. During those years major refinements had been made in the design and safety of balloon catheters.

Pulmonary valvuloplasty and pulmonary valve stenosis: The clinical profile of pulmonary valve stenosis had been known since the 1950's and auscultatory and electrocardiographic assessment of severity were reliable, though less precise than later obtained with Doppler echocardiography. Brock had described succesful closed heart surgery for pulmonic stenosis in 1948 [106]; later, in the early 1950's surgery using hypothermia without cardiopulmonary bypass had been performed [159]. In 1961 Brock described pulmonary valvulotomy with a valvulotome introduced through a small ventriculotomy, followed by a Hegar dilator. This led to great optimism on the feasibility of dilatation without surgery.

Despite the obvious attractions of catheter dilatation as a concept, the management of a stenotic pulmonary valve was already highly successful by 1982. The Natural History Study [171]. and observations from many centers had shown three important points: when pulmonary valvar stenosis was mild, with a right ventricular to pulmonary artery pressure gradient of 25mm/Hg or less, it very rarely progressed, and these children required no treatment and led normal lives: when open heart surgery was needed, the results were excellent, with almost no operative mortality if performed beyond infancy; morbidity was minor, chiefly from postpericardiotomy syndrome: postoperative recurrence was highly unusual and endocarditis almost non-existent. Later follow up of the same group of patients in 6 major heart centers, using agreed criteria of medical or surgical management, had survival rates over 25 years or more virtually indistinguishable from that of individuals born with normal hearts. Thus it required great courage to introduce a new method of treatment. This courage has been rewarded by the test of time. Patients, families and physicians have all found the brevity of the procedure, the absence of anesthesia or scar on the chest, and the need for only a few hours of hospitalistion, to be great assets of pulmonary valvuloplasty. It is clearly here to stay, and the risk of recurrence has been found to be minimal, even lower than that following surgery.

Although a relatively common defect, present in approximately 9% of live born infants with heart defects, it seldom needs treatment in early infancy. An otherwise healthy infant with a harsh pulmonary ejection murmur can now have a definitive echocardiographic diagnosis made at any age: the family can be reassured that surgical intervention will be unnecessary. The frequency of ambulatory follow up varies with severity, but is usually at yearly intervals. If and when pulmonary valvuloplasty is needed, even an overnight stay in the hospital can often be avoided, and no further catheterisations will be needed. This overall coherent plan avoids hospitalisation, radiation exposure (except for the one catheter intervention), and any tinge of invalidism. Now practiced world wide, the only problems appear to be with dysplastic valves, typical of Noonan syndrome but occasionally seen in otherwise normal children.

Interventional cardiology: The dramatic story of pulmonary valvuloplasty led to a search for other uses of what came to be known as invasive or interventional cardiology. The establishment of a VACA Registry in 1982 helped to standardise techniques and indications for both pulmonary and aortic valvuloplasty. The role of balloon dilatation in other defects such as native coarctation, fibromuscular subaortic membrane, and peripheral pulmonic stenosis continues to be assessed. Balloon dilatation has also been used in rheumatic mitral stenosis, particularly in Third World countries where this remains a common problem. Numerically, the number of angioplasties for atherosclerotic coronary artery disease far exceeds the total balloon dilatations for congenital defects, and indeed this technique, pioneered by Gruentzig in 1978 [243], has provided a whole new invasive world for the cardiologist working with adults.

Other invasive techniques found useful in occasional infants or children include balloons or coils for closure of pulmonary arteriovenous malformations or the large aortopulmonary collaterals which may complicate tetralogy with pulmonary atresia. In the scimitar syndrome, closures of the massive aberrant artery from the descending aorta to the right lower lobe of the lung has been successful in abolishing intractable heart failure. The rarity and technical difficulty of such applications is a strong argument for them to be done in only a few centers.

Tools or devices for closing atrial or ventricular septal defects or patent ductus differ greatly from the concept of pulmonary valvuloplasty. All such devices require the introduction and permanent placement of foreign material in the cardiovascular system. It is too soon to know what role, if any, such devices will play in the future of pediatric cardiology [177,244-246].

Other Heart Problems in Infants and Children

During the years between the mid 1970s and 1990, Kawasaki syndrome, cardiomyopathy, and arrhythmias began to receive much attention from pediatric cardiologists. Kawasaki syndrome alone seems to have been newly described; cardiomyopathy and arrhythmias had always been recognised, but in the absence of many of the modern tools of diagnosis and follow up, had received little attention.

KAWASAKI SYNDROME

Following the original description by Kawasaki in 1967, mucocutaneous lymph node syndrome shortly thereafter was reported in Europe [247], the United States, and around the world. Myocarditis and pericardial effusion may complicate the acute phase, but the major reason for cardiologic concern is the coronary artery dilatation and aneurysms which can occur, and lead occasionally to late sudden death. The syndrome aroused intense anxiety in parents and physicians alike in the early years, because of the apparent unpredictability of its course, the initial difficulty in adequate visualisation of the coronary arteries on echocardiography, and the uncertainty regarding treatment.

Kawasaki syndrome can now be said to be a disorder which represents a triumph of collaborative clinical research. The pathogenesis is still being studied, some authorities maintaining a viral etiology, others implicating a streptococcal superantigen. Collaborative treatment trials have conclusively shown the value of gamma globulin infusion early in the course of the illness in preventing the later development of coronary artery aneurysms. Although the disease itself is not yet preventable, the sequelae, with very rare exceptions, are. This is one of the rare conditions where the future role of the cardiologist should in most cases be a minor one; since the illness will be managed, except for any echocardiography indicated, by the primary care physician. The American Heart Association has recently issued guidelines for risk stratification and long term management [248].

From a historical point of view, at least two questions arise: "How much of current coronary artery disease in young adults is caused by prior unrecognised Kawasaki syndrome?" and "Is it really a new disease, or one misdiagnosed or unrecognised in the past?" In the last twenty years of unceasing coronary arteriography at Johns Hopkins, there seems to have been only one young adult whose findings were compatible with prior Kawasaki involvement, which suggests this sequel is a rare phenomenon. The second question has been much debated; it is true that diagnosis of the acute illness can at times be confusing, and in the pre-echocardiographic era, unruptured coronary artery aneurysms would not have been detected. Richard Rowe and Vera Rose [249], in an autopsy study at the Hospital for Sick Children in Toronto, found coronary aneurysms present in children before the syndrome was described, and postulated that in the past, such children had been diagnosed to have atypical measles.

Whether or not Kawasaki is a new disease of childhood, we have observed it sweep into history, become diagnosable, and yield to early treatment, all within a span of thirty years. Can this be said of any other illness?

CARDIOMYOPATHY

Certainly childhood cardiomyopathy has not followed the exhilarating course of Kawasaki disease. New causes are recognised with increasing frequency, a number of them iatrogenic, as in anthracycline toxicity or the myocardial hypertrophy seen after long term steroid therapy.

When the term cardiomyopathy was first introduced [153], the concept was to exclude myocardial disease secondary to congenital defects, systemic hypertension, or coronary atherosclerosis. This concept was very helpful in defining the important group of primary disorders of heart muscle, and thus allowing cardiomyopathy to be categorised and studied. There has now appeared a small but distressing group of patients who began life with a congenital cardiac defect, underwent one or more operative procedures, and now have hearts which are anatomically corrected, but exhibit profound myocardial dysfunction. Some of these have responded well to cardiac transplantation, others have not had this option. This small "secondary" group now exists in addition to a burgeoning number of causes of primary cardiomyopathy in childhood.

Myocarditis of non rheumatic origin began to be discussed in the pediatric literature in the early 1940's [250]. The term "Fiedler's myocarditis" was still occasionally used, because in 1899 Fiedler had described some of the pathologic findings of acute myocardial inflammation [206a]. In the 1950's, about the time that identification of specific viral causes of disease became possible, there were a number of papers on Coxsackie myocarditis in the neonate. One of the features which aroused great interest was that a mild viral illness in thè mother was associated with a very high perinatal mortality.

Long before this time, diphtheria was a deadly disease of childhood. Many of the deaths were due to respiratory obstruction, and pediatricians in the early years of this century needed to have tracheostomy skills in their armamentarium. Some of the mortality was due to acute fatty infiltration of the myocardium produced by the diphtheria toxin. The pathology has been well described, and is a toxic rather than an inflammatory type of myocardial damage. Recently it has been suggested that the diphtheria toxin acts by depletion of carnitine. It is likely that pediatric cardiologists were not much drawn to discuss or write about this phenomenon because by the time pediatric cardiology began, in the early 1940's, diphtheria immunisation had essentially abolished the disease in the USA and Western Europe. John Nihoyannopolous, one of Helen Taussig's best loved former Fellows, returned from Athens to a Clinic Reunion in the early 1960's, and presented some findings of children with post diphtheritic heart block and arrhythmias. Others at the Reunion, at that time completely absorbed in the intricacies of structural heart disease and the triumphs of surgery, felt such matters were only for the Greeks. Few, if any, recognised that cardiomyopathy and arrhythmias would soon be among the major topics at all gatherings of pediatric cardiologists.

Early descriptions of pediatric viral myocarditis, of presumed or (rarely) proven etiology, focused on recognition by electrocardiographic criteria. A number of studies showed some electrocardiographic changes during the course of many of the childhood exanthemata, including chickenpox and measles, leading to the concept that subclinical myocardial inflammation was not infrequent in childhood viral illness. The electrocardiographic differentiation from endocardial fibroelastosis of infancy was a major theme in the 1950's and early 1960's. (The essential disappearance of endocardial fibroelastosis is one of the minor, but pleasing, mysteries of the history of pediatric cardiology). It was not until the mid 1960's that pediatric cardiologists really awoke to the poor prognosis of many infants and children, and the long term sequel of dilated cardiomyopathy. The controversies surrounding the role and timing of cardiac biopsy in myocarditis, the indications for immunosuppressive therapy including gammaglobulin infusion, and the methods of stratifying risk factors, are too large a topic to embark on here. Some valuable collaborative studies are underway, exploring the concept that early and vigorous treatment of acute myocarditis in a child or adult may prevent the later ravages of dilated cardiomyopathy.

Since the mid 1970's echocardiographic techniques have provided a method of following ventricular size and function during the acute and recovery phases. Prior to the echocardiogram, all other tools for attempted monitoring were unreliable. As research on myocarditis and dilated cardiomyopathy has intensified, the advent of cardiac transplantation has also spurred awareness of the primary role of the normal myocardium in childhood heart health.

Cardiomyopathy, dilated, hypertrophic and restrictive. The classification of cardiomyopathy into these three types was introduced by John Goodwin and his colleagues in a series of communications dating from 1960 [153], and was later adopted by WHO. As each etiologic subgroup is teased out of the complex of heart muscle disorders, it is clear that some, such as carnitine deficiency, may cross boundaries and result in dilated cardiomyopathy in some children and the hypertrophic form in others. Nevertheless, the classification is of great value clinically at all ages.

Dilated cardiomyopathy was brought to the attention of pediatricians in the United States in 1984 by Marjorie Tripp [251]. The most frequent etiology in children, as in adults, is a prior viral illness. Metabolic causes include carnitine deficiency, which may in turn be either environmental or due to a recessive metabolic defect. The list of possible causes is lengthening, but anthracycline toxicity is among the most frequent etiologies seen in children's centers. It is likely, though unproven, that AIDS infection, exacerbated by nutritional deficiencies, is now the major etiology in children worldwide. In cardiac centers the role of medications, including angiotensin inhibitors and anticoagulants, and the timing of cardiac transplantation, are still evolving. Although no doubt present throughout recorded time, the history of dilated cardiomyopathy in childhood began as a concept in 1960; its history lies in the future, still to be written.

Hypertrophic cardiomyopathy was known to pediatrics in one of its rarest manifestations from 1933, when Pompe [252] described the form of glycogen storage disease of the heart later found to be due to deficiency of the enzyme acid alpha 1,4-glucosidase. This was approximately 30 years before the term cardiomyopathy was coined. Despite its extreme rarity, the entity was much discussed because of the specific electrocardiographic pattern of a short PR interval and left ventricular hypertrophy, and because of recessive mode of inheritance. It is now often included in discussions of "metabolic" or genetic forms of cardiomyopathy [253].

The disorder most usually thought of as representing hypertrophic cardiomyopathy was described by Teare in 1958. There had been earlier reports by Bernheim and others of massive unexplained ventricular hypertrophy, but Teare's report is of particular interest both for the terminology of his title, and for the later follow up [254, 255]. The term he used, "asymmetric hypertrophy," has worn well, and familial asymmetric septal hypertrophy is now a condition recognised worldwide.

Barry Maron [256], who acquired a unique perspective on the familial syndrome during his years at the National Institutes of Health working with Stanley Epstein and Glenn Morrow, has emphasised the many synonyms used by different groups. For a number of years British cardiologists favored HOCM (hypertrophic obstructive cardiomyopathy), partly at least because they liked the sound and implication of "hokum," obscure and a little tricky. They were undeterred by the fact that actual outflow obstruction was relatively infrequent. The disorder was early recognised to be familial, inherited by an autosomal dominant mode of transmission. The distinctive clinical findings of a brisk pulse upstroke, marked left ventricular hypertrophy, and a significant risk of sudden death were all reported prior to the widespread use of echocardiography.

The Doppler echocardiogram has been valuable, both in genetic studies, and in confirming that the underlying physiologic problem is usually one of ventricular filling rather than outflow obstruction [257]. Despite the use of calcium channel blockers and selective surgical intervention, there is little evidence that the clinical course of the disorder has been greatly improved. Recent genetic studies have shown mutations in the beta-myosin heavy chain located on chromosome 14.

The sequence of progress in knowledge, from anatopathologic description, through clinicophysiologic correlation to recognition in infancy, and now to molecular biology, is thus very similar to that for structural heart disease, though the history has been more abbreviated and the therapy less dramatic.

Other forms of hypertrophic cardiomyopathy seen in childhood include those in neuromuscular diseases such as Duchenne muscular dystrophy, and Noonan among other syndromes.

Restrictive cardiomyopathy in children was originally described as endomyocardial fibrosis, confined chiefly to Africa. It is now recognised to occur worldwide, being usually known as hypereosinophilic endomyocardial disease. It is seen less frequently than the other forms, and has a poor prognosis often requiring early cardiac transplantation.

Arrhythmogenic right ventricle is among the many other cardiomyopathy variants that are being identified and studied. Although the history of cardiomyopathies in childhood appears brief, this must be attributed to lack of recognition in early years of high childhood mortality and lack of modern tools of cardiac evaluation. In all forms, growth of knowledge has been rapid, and followed the general outline shown in Figure 1, but treatment and prevention are still elusive.

PEDIATRIC ARRHYTHMIAS: ELECTROCARDIOGRAPHY IN CHILDREN

It may seem inappropriate to include a sketch of Willem Einthoven (Figure 13), who died in 1927, in a chapter on the infant era of pediatric cardiology, which began in the mid 1970's. We have done so to dramatise the continuity of history. The tool of the electrocardiogram dates from 1902, and most of the present concepts of arrhythmias and electrical spatial vectors had evolved by the mid 1950's. However, pediatric arrhythmias did not become a focus of attention until the infant era.

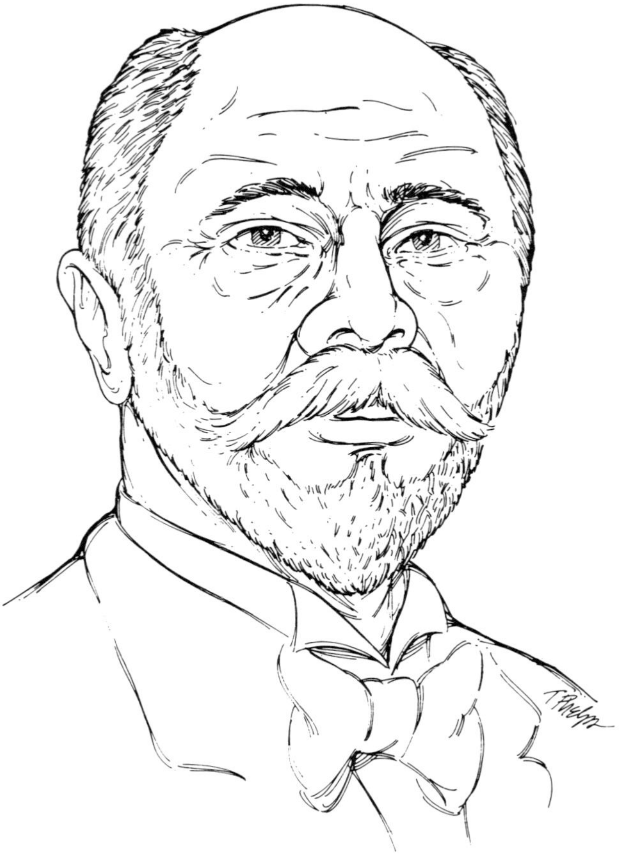

Figure 13. Willem Einthoven (1860-1927), of Leiden, inventor of the electrocardiogram.

Bruce Fye has written an absorbing account of the history of arrhythmias [258], and the evolution of scientific thinking which led to the recognition and naming of most rhythm disorders by the middle of this century. In his study of the history of electrocardiography [11], he also reviews the impact this new tool had on medicine, including its important role in defining cardiology as a specialty. Fye describes how Einthoven circumvented the problems inherent in his "massive 600 pound apparatus," the string galvanometer for recording electrocardiograms, by using a telephone cable to transmit the electrical impulses from the hearts of hospitalised patients to his laboratory over a mile away [11,79]. It was to be almost 80 years before telemetry was widely used in studying arrhythmias in the young.

The electrocardiogram spread from Leiden throughout the world, became portable, and became of use in the diagnosis at first of cardiac arrhythmias and later of myocardial infarction. This brief summary is not intended to convey the depth and scholarship of Fye's analysis, but rather to use it as a basis for discussing the rather different, much later, course followed in pediatric cardiology.

Fye comments that in the early 1920's the electrocardiogram was already in widespread clinical use, and a patient with heart disease often had an electrocardiographic tracing in his possession. Patients then, as now, clearly enjoyed technology. (One cannot help wondering when and how this excellent habit of a patient bearing portable recorded data disappeared).

As pediatric cardiology began to emerge as a discipline in the 1940's, electrocardiograms were taken on all patients coming for evaluation. There was a separate room for electrocardiography, the precursor of the much larger and more elaborate Pediatric Heart Station of later decades; the studies were stored and available for future research. There were a few communications on supraventricular tachycardia and on congenital heart block in the early 1950's and 1960's [181,259,260], but the focus was on using the electrocardiogram as a tool in the diagnosis of structural heart defects [114,117]. Wolff, Parkinson and White had described their syndrome in 1930 [261], but the important role of preexcitation in rhythm disorders in the young was not yet recognised. Only later, in the 1970's, did the focus of attention turn to arrhythmias. In this section we will briefly explore this sequence, the early electrocardiograms, the growth of interest in arrhythmias, and the current use of electrocardiographic tools.

Early electrocardiograms in children were used to establish normal rates, intervals and voltages at different ages [111,112]. In the early years, arrhythmias were poorly recognised in children and were thought to be mostly benign. Electrocardiographic monitoring was in its infancy, and it was not until the 1970s that the frequency of neonatal arrhythmias was appreciated. In the 1950's, even after the advent of closed heart surgery, postoperative arrhythmias were seldom encountered. The electrocardiogram was used mainly as a tool of clinical diagnosis. Great interest was aroused by the diagnostic patterns seen in Ebstein anomaly, tricuspid atresia, and atrioventricular septal defects [115,117,262]. Although measurement of the QT interval had been described in 1952, it was to be many years before the long QT syndrome was defined [181].

Empiric observations had confirmed Sodi-Pollares' claim [118] of the characteristic sequence of ventricular activation in tetralogy of Fallot, one of the main areas of interest. The very small number of papers written on the preoperative EKG in tetralogy attests to the commonly held view that when you had seen one, you had seen them all. While this was an exaggeration, the lack of arrhythmias pre or postoperatively while only shunt procedures were being done could not be denied. Robert Ziegler of Detroit [111] and John Keith of Toronto [206] were among the few who made a systematic study of the electrocardiogram prior to the era of open heart surgery. Jerry Liebman later pioneered in the use of the vectorcardiogram as providing an analytic approach to the hypertrophy patterns seen in malformed hearts [262].

By the beginning of open heart surgery in 1955, most of the diagnostic patterns had already been described, including the remarkable infarct pattern seen in anomalous origin of the left coronary from the pulmonary artery. Increasingly the electrocardiogram was used as an indicator of physiology, and in assessing non invasively the severity of pulmonary valve stenosis or ventricular septal defect [171]. The dawn of open heart surgery brought many challenges, among them the recognition that postoperative arrhythmias might be frequent and severe, and that new electrocardiographic patterns, particularly right bundle branch block, often followed ventriculotomy. Although pediatric cardiologists and surgeons were aware of the course of the conducting system when open heart surgery began, the knowledge was to become much more vivid and urgent shortly thereafter, once a surgical needle or stitch might encroach on that structure with a seemingly historic name, the bundle of His.

Arryhthmias began to be studied in the 1960's, stimulated in part by the needs in postoperative care, and in part by increasing interest in cardiac physiology. One of the first collaborative studies concerned **congenital heart block** [263]. The prognosis was known to be variable, some patients dying in infancy, others leading normal lives for many years. The problem was sufficiently rare that no one center could establish the true natural history. Cardiac pacemakers had been introduced in the late 1950's [181], and one stimulus for this international study was to determine if any specific ventricular rate or other sign indicated that a pacemaker was needed. The association of heart block with maternal connective tissue diseases was reported in 1977 by Carolyn McCue and her group [264]; a few years later the etiology was established, the passage of maternal Ro antibodies across the conducting system to attack the developing conducting system.

The malignant course of surgically induced complete heart block was recognised early, and new surgical techniques swiftly made it a very rare problem.

In 1952 Alexander Nadas [259] had described the clinical course of 41 infants and children with **supraventricular tachycardia**. Paroxysmal tachycardia had been described late in the 19th century, and named by Sir Thomas Lewis in 1909 [258]. But Nadas' paper was among the first to draw attention to a condition which could prove lethal in a previously healthy infant. It began the process, which grew remarkably in later decades during the infant era, of clarifying in what respects pediatric arrhythmias differed from those already well recognised in adults. His communication stressed the young age of onset and the risk of recurrence within the first year of life, points confirmed by many subsequent writers. At first digoxin with or without quinidine were the only form of treatment.

John Keith, in 1967, used his Toronto heart registry data base to calculate the prevalence of paroxysmal supraventricular tachycardia in children as 1/25,000.

By 1981, when Garson and associates [265] described 217 children with the condition seen over a period of 25 years, they considered Keith's figure to be possibly an underestimate. By 1981, several differences from Nadas' report of 30 years earlier had emerged. Many more medications were now in use, and cardioversion and overdrive pacing had been adapted for pediatric patients. Postoperative arrhythmias were now adding to the population studied; twenty three children, more than 10% of their group, had had prior intracardiac surgery, usually a Mustard procedure. The wide range of treatment options for this usually benign condition was producing a considerable degree of controversy and confusion; fortunately, the introduction of adenosine as the drug of choice in the late 1980's transformed the approach to most acute episodes of supraventricular tachycardia in the young.

The high frequency and progressive nature of **other atrial arrhythymias** following intratrial procedures for transposition acted as a further stimulus to pathologic [266] and electrophysiologic [267] studies of the sinus node. Although electrophysiologic studies added little to the basic concepts of electrocardiography, by their precision and reproducibility they undoubtedly laid the groundwork for future surgical [268] and catheter [269] treatment of refractory arrhythmias.

The assumption that premature ventricular contractions were always benign in the pediatric age group came under suspicion with the recognition of sudden death in occasional young patients with hypertrophic cardiomyopathy, long QT syndrome [270], and as a late complication following open tetralogy repair [271].

The work of Paul Gillette and Arthur (Tim) Garson, both formerly of Houston, beginning in the infant era, brought a new, systematic, and vigorous approach to the diagnosis and therapy of pediatric arrhythmias [181].

It is interesting to look back on the early recordings of Einthoven, before he developed his string galvanometer (Figure 14), and reflect on how much has grown, for adults and children alike, from his discovery.

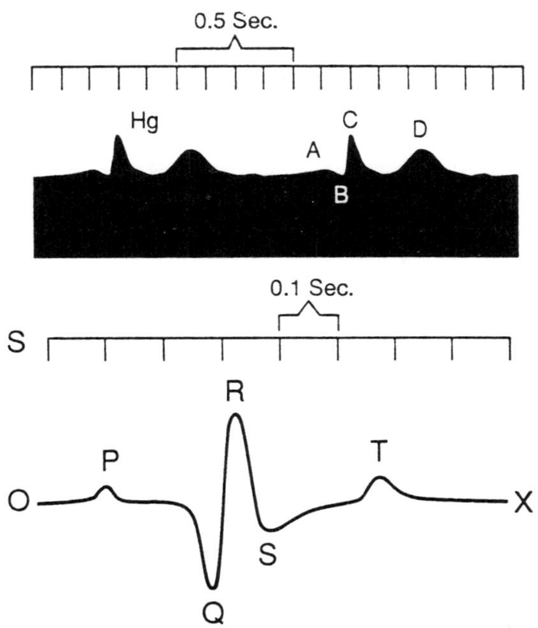

Figure 14 Precursors of the electrocardiogram: recorded by Einthoven before his first electrocardiographic recording with the string galvanometer. "Great oaks from little acorns grow." Modified with permission from Fishman and Richards 1964 [5].

Electrocardiographic tools now available in the 1990's have changed dramatically since the time of Einthoven. Ambulatory monitoring (introduced in 1961), electrophysiologic studies, new medications, and transcatheter ablation of aberrant pathways [269] are all now in daily use for those with severe arrhythmias. Collaborative studies of affected families are revealing the molecular basis of the long QT syndrome. Table 4 records a few of the memorable dates in rhythm disturbances of childhood.

Table 4
Some Memorable Dates in Childhood Arrhythmia [181, 258]

1890	Morquio	Familial heart block
1902	Einthoven	Electrocardiogram using string galvanometer
1930	WPW	Wolff Parkinson White syndrome
1952	Nadas	SVT in children
1957	Jervell Lange-Nielsen	Prolonged QT with sudden death
1972	Collaborative study	Complete heart block
1975-1990		Long QT syndrome: cardioversion: antiarrhythmic drugs: ventricular arrhythmias: family studies: ambulatory monitoring: exercise testing: EPS
1991	Collaborative study	Radiofrequency catheter ablation

It is likely that there were earlier accounts of rhythm disturbances in the young than shown in this table. The table is not intended to be comprehensive, but simply to highlight the great changes in tools and concepts devoted to pediatric arrhythmia in the fifteen years of the infant era, 1975 to 1990.

With the advent of echocardiography, the role of the electrocardiogram in the analysis of structural anomalies or physiologic change has lessened from 40 years ago. But its role has increased exponentially in arrhythmia detection, and in the evaluation of which arrhythmias can be abolished with medication or invasive therapy. Postoperative arrhythmias are decreasing with improved myocardial preservation and younger age at surgery; "new" causes of arrhythmias include self administered cardiotoxins such as cocaine and crack, and prescribed medications including psychotropic drugs. Einthoven's tool of the electrocardiogram continues to find new uses in the care of childrens' hearts.

Preventive Cardiology

By the mid 1980's research from many sources showed that much adult cardiac disease has its origins in childhood. Studies of coronary artery risk factors in children, including diet, exercise, heredity, and blood pressure, involving children in Muscatine, Iowa [272], Bogalusa, Louisiana [273], and Rochester, Minnesota [274] were begun in the decades of the 1950's to 1970's and most are still ongoing. The concept of primary prevention of atherosclerosis, or preventive cardiology [275], is now part of the mainstream of pediatric cardiac literature [276]. These concepts have emerged from use of many tools, including epidemiologic research [277,278], biochemical lipoprotein analysis [279], and genetic linkage studies. Although unanimity has not been reached [280] on the best approach to preserving the healthy heart of a child, there is an emerging concept that cardiac health is a continuum affected by both genetic and environmental factors, and is a major domain of pediatric cardiology.

Two Young Women with Palpitations

We have tried to end each chapter with a passage conveying the concept that cardiac history involves young people and their families in the world outside medical academia. Although this chapter deals with the infant era, we have chosen two stories of young adults with arrhythmias. One of these young women is fictional, the other a living modern poet. The story of the first will be used to consider, in a light hearted way, the progress in arrhythmias over the past 100 years. The words of the second will be quoted, as a relief from medical prose.

CHECKOV AND THE COUNTRY DOCTOR

The date is approximately 1880. The short story, entitled "A Doctors Visit" is included in On Doctoring edited by Richard Reynolds and John Stone published by Simon and Schuster New York 1991. The young Dr Korolyov visits the 20 year old daughter of a prominent factory owner, two railroad stations and a coach drive from Moscow. On his way into the sickroom, the governess, Christina Dmitryevna, tells the doctor that Liza has been ailing from a child. "The doctors say it is nerves; when she was a little girl she was scrofulous, and the doctors drove it inwards, so I think it may be due to that." After this, Dr Korolyov proceeds to see his patient, whom he could hardly believe was the heiress of the five large buidings on the estate: ...

> *"I have palpitations of the heart," she said. "It was so awful all night ... I almost died of fright! Do give me something."*
>
> *"I will, I will, don't worry yourself."*
>
> *Korolyov examined her and shrugged his shoulders.*
>
> *"The heart is all right," he said, "... everything is in good order ... The attack is over by now, one must suppose; lie down and go to sleep." ...*

The mother, Madame Lyalikov, to her daughter
"Lizanka, you are crying again . . . again . . . Tell me what it is!" Both wept bitterly.
Korolyov sat down by the side of the bed and took Liza's hand.
"Come, give over, its no use crying," he said kindly . . . And inwardly he thought:
"Its high time she was married . . ."

The Doctor's Visit by Anton Chekhov from The Lady with the Dog and Other Stories copyright Macmillan 1972 published Ecco Press 1984. Excerpted with permission.

It is interesting to speculate on the different diagnoses offered to this young Russian woman, who herself believed her symptoms heralded approaching death. Her governess, a slightly ambivalent observer, diagnosed scrofula turned inwards, a diagnosis no longer favored in our times. The physician clearly believes that the diagnosis was psychosomatic, and that the best cure would be the advent of a significant other, preferably of a marriageable disposition. He was neither the first nor the last to hold this opinion, and across the distance of time and fiction we cannot prove him wrong.

We have chosen to speculate that the patient was having episodes of supraventricular tachycardia due to Wolff Parkinson White syndrome. If she lived another 20 years she could have an electrocardiogram; by 1909, Sir Thomas Lewis in London had described paroxysmal tachycardia [258], and might have treated her with digitalis. Only if she slept, like Sleeping Beauty, for the next 100 years, could she have woken in 1985 in an electrophysiologic laboratory to have ablation of her aberrant pathway. Did she have a bundle of Kent, or of Tashkent?

The second young woman is a Canadian poet, Margaret Atwood, who wrote a poem "The Woman Who Could Not Live With Her Faulty Heart," excerpted below with permission:

"But most hearts say, I want, I want,
I want, I want. My heart
is more duplicitous,
though no twin as I once thought.
It says, I want, I dont want, I
want, and then a pause.
It forces me to listen . . .

Long ago I gave up singing
to it, it will never be satisfied or lulled.
One night I will say to it:
Heart, be still,
and it will."

Margaret Atwood "The woman who could not live with her faulty heart," copyright Houghton Mifflin 1987 Selected Poems II. Selected Poems 1966-1984 Oxford U Press 1990 copyright M. Atwood excerpted with permission.

ADDITIONAL REFERENCES AND NOTES

205. Rowe RD, Mehrizi A. The Neonate with Congenital Heart Disease. Philadelphia. WB Saunders, 1968.

206. Keith JD. Prevalence, incidence and epidemiology. In: Keith JD, Rowe RD, Vlad P editors Heart disease in infancy and childhood. 3rd ed. New York: Macmillan 1978:3-13.

206a. Myocarditis ibid 1978:926-940.

207. Kan JS, White RI Jr., Mitchell SE, Gardner TJ. Percutaneous balloon valvuloplasty: a new method of treating congenital pulmonary valve stenosis. New Eng J Med 1982;307:540-542.

208. Anderson PAW. Physiology of the fetal, neonatal and adult heart. In: Fetal and Neonatal Physiology. Polin RA, Fox WW, editors. Philadelphia: WB Saunders 1992: 722-758.

209. Lurie PR, Fujito M, Neustein HB. Transvascular endomyocardial biopsy in infants and small children: description of a new technique. Am J Cardiol 1978;42:452-453.

210. Clark E, Takao A editors. Developmental cardiology: Morphogenesis and function. Mount Kisco NY: Futura 1990.

211. Kirby ML, Gale TF, Stewart DE. Neural crest cells contribute to normal aortico-pulmonary septation. Science 1983;220:1059-1061.

212. Clark EB. Mechanisms in the pathogenesis of congenital cardiac malformations. In: Pierpont MEM, Moller JH, editors. Genetics of Cardiovascular Disease. Boston, Martinius Nijhoff 1986:3-11.

213. Emanuel R, Somerville J, Inns A, Withers R. Evidence of congenital heart disease in the offspring of parents with atrioventricular septal defects. Brit Heart J 1983;49:144-147.

214. Pyeritz RE, Murphy EA. Genetics and congenital heart disease: Perspectives and prospects. J Am Coll Cardiol 1989;13:1458-1468.

215. Burn J, Richards SJ, Brennan P, Wyse RKH. Molecular genetic strategies in the investigation of congenital heart malformations. In: Clark EB, Takao A editors. Developmental Cardiology: Morphogenesis and Function. Mount Kisco NY Futura 1990;557-571.

216. Dietz HC, Cutting GR, Pyeritz RE, Maslen CL, et al. Marfan syndrome caused by a recurrent de novo missense mutation in the fibrillin gene. Nature 1991;352:337-339.

217. Ferencz C, Rubin JD, Loffredo CA, Magee CA. Epidemiology of Congenital Heart Disease: The Baltimore-Washington Infant Study 1981-1989. Perspectives in Pediatric Cardiology. Anderson RH, series editor. Mount Kisco NY: Futura 1993.

218. Blumenthal S. Foreword. In: Congenital cardiac defects-recent advances. Birth Defects Original Article Series. Baltimore, Wiliams and Wilkins for March of Dimes 1972;8:1.

219. Ultan LB, Segal BL, Likoff W. Echocardiography in congenital heart disease. preliminary observations. Am J Cardiol 1967;19:74-83.

220. The Johns Hopkins Medical Journal: An issue dedicated to Helen B. Taussig. Johns Hopkins Med J 1977;140:143-205.

221. Elliott RB, Starling MB, Neutze JM. Medical manipulation of the ductus arteriosus. Lancet 1975;1:140-142.

222. Olley PM, Coceani F, Bodach E. E-type prostaglandins: A new emergency therapy for certain cyanotic congenital heart malformations. Circulation 1976;53:728-731.

223. Friedman WF, Hirschklau MJ, Printz MP Pittick PT, Kirkpatrick SE. Pharmacologic closure of patent ductus arteriosus in the premature infant. New Eng J Med 1976;295: 526-528.

224. Barratt-Boyes BG, Neutze JM, Clarkson PM, Shardey GC, Brandt PWT. Repair of ventricular septal defect in the first two years of life using profound hypothermia and total circulatory arrest techniques. Ann Surg 1976;184:376-390.

225. Castaneda AR, Freed MD, Williams RG, Norwood WI. Repair of tetralogy of Fallot in infancy. Early and late results. J Thorac Cardiovasc Surg 1977;74:372-381.

226. Macartney FJ, Taylor JFN, Graham GR, De Leval M, Stark J. The fate of survivors of cardiac surgery in infancy. Circulation 1980; 62:80-91.

227. Norwood WI, Lang P, Hansen DD. Physiologic repair of aortic atresia-hypoplastic left heart syndrome. New Eng J Med 1983;308:23-26.

228. Cameron DE, Gardner TJ. Heart transplantation in children. In: Heart and heart lung transplantation, Baumgartner WA, Reitz BA, Achuff SC editors. Philadelphia: WB Saunders, 1990:293-302.

229. Jatene AD, Fontes VF, Paulista PP, Souza LCB et al. Anatomic correction of transposition of the great vessels. J Thorac Cardiovasc Surg 1976;72:364-370.

230. Castaneda AR, Trusler GA, Paul MH, Blackstone EH, Kirklin JW, Congenital Heart Surgeons Society. The early results of treatment of simple transposition in the current era. J Thorac Cardiovasc Surg 1988;95:14-28.

231. Lecompte Y, Zannini L, Hazan E, Jarreau MM, et al. Anatomic correction of transposition of the great arteries. A new technique without use of a prosthetic conduit. J Thorac Cardiovasc Surg 1981;82:629-631.

232. Planche C, Bruniaux J, Lacour-Gayet F, Kachaner J, et al. Switch operation for transposition of the great arteries in neonates. A study of 120 patients. J Thorac Cardiovasc Surg 1988;96:354-363.

233. Neill CA, Clark EB, Clark C. The Heart of a Child. Baltimore:Johns Hopkins Press 1992.

234. Kirklin JW. The movement of cardiac surgery to the very young. In: Perspectives in Pediatric Cardiology. Vol 2 Pediatric Cardiac Surgery Part 1. Crupi G, Parenzan L, Anderson RH, editors. Mount Kisco NY: Futura 1989:3-20.

235. Frescura C, Thiene G, Franceschini E, Talenti E, Mazzucco A. Pulmonary vascular disease in infants with complete atrioventricular septal defect. Int J Cardiol 1987;15:91-100.

236. Freedom RM, Bini M, Rowe RD. Endocardial cushion defect and significant hypoplasia of the left ventricle: a distinct clinical and pathological entity. Eur J Cardiol 1978;7:263-281.

237. Kallen B. Population surveillance of multimalformed infants-experience with the Swedish Registry of Congenital Malformations. J Genet Humain 1987;35:321-338.

238. Pieroni DR, Homcy E, Freedom RM. Echocardiography in atrioventricular canal defect. A clinical spectrum. Am J Cardiol 1975;35:54-58.

239. Bom N, Lancee CT, Zwieten GV, Kloster FE, Roelandt J. Multiscan echocardiography I. Technical description. Circulation 1973;48:1066-1074.

240. Snider RA, Serwer GA. Echocardiography in pediatric heart disease Chicago: Year Book Med Publishers 1990.

241. Allan LD, Tynan MJ, Campbell S, Wilkinson JL, Anderson RH. Echocardiographic and anatomic correlates in the fetus. Brit Heart J 1980;44:444-451.

242. Cook AC, Allan LD, Anderson RH, Sharland G, Fagg NLK. Atrioventricular septal defect in fetal life-a clinicopathological correlation. Cardiology in the Young 1991;1:334-343.

243. Gruentzig A. Transluminal dilatation of coronary artery stenosis. Lancet 1978;1:263.

244. Rashkind WJ, Wagner HR, Tait MA. Historical perspectives of interventional cardiology: Past, present and future. Texas Heart Inst J 1986;13:363-367.

245. Report of the European Registry. Transcatheter occlusion of the persistent arterial duct. Lancet 1992;340:1062-1066.

246. Castaneda AR, Jonas RA, Mayer JE Jr., Hanley FL. Cardiac surgery of the neonate and infant. Philadelphia: WB Saunders 1994.

247. Della Porta G, Alberti A. Kawasaki disease in Europe. Lancet 1977;1:797-798.

248. Dajani AS, Taubert KA, Takahashi M, Bierman FZ et al. Guidelines for long term management of patients with Kawasaki disease. Circulation 1994;89:916-922.

249. Rowe P. Personal comunication 1994.

250. Saphir O, Wile SA, Reingold IM. Myocarditis in children. Am J Dis Child 1944;67:294-312.

251. Tripp M. Congestive cardiomyopathy of childhood. Adv Ped 1984;31:179-206.

252. Pompe JD. Over idiopatische hypertrophy van het hart. Nederl Tijdschr Geneesk 1932;76:304-306. Also Hypertrophie idiopathique du coeur Ann Anat Path 1933;10:23-24.

253. Kohlschutter A, Hausdorf G. Primary (genetic) cardiomyopathies in infancy. A survey of possible disorders and guidelines for diagnosis. Eur J Ped 1986;145:454-459.

254. Teare D. Asymmetrical hypertrophy of the heart in young patients. Brit Heart J 1958;20:1-8.

255. Watkins H, Seidman CE, MacRae C, Seidman JG, McKenna W. Progress in familial hypertrophic cardiomyopathy: molecular genetic analyses in the original family studied by Teare. Brit Heart J 1992;67:34-38.

256. Maron BJ, Tajik AJ, Ruttenburg HD et al. Hypertrophic cardiomyopathy in infants: clinical features and natural history. Circulation 1982;65:7-17.

257. Gidding SS, Snider AR, Rocchini AP et al. Left ventricular diastolic filling in children with hypertrophic cardiomyopathy: assessment with pulsed Doppler echocardiography. J Am Coll Cardiol 1986;8:310-316.

258. Fye WB. Disorders of the heart beat—A historical overview from antiquity to the mid 20th century. Am J Cardiol 1993;72:1055-1070.

259. Nadas AS, Doeschner GW, Roth A, Blumenthal SL. Paroxysmal tachycardia in infants and children. Study of 41 cases. Pediatrics 1952;9:167-173.

260. Landtmann B, Linder E, Hjelt L et al. Congenital complete heart block. I. A clinical study of 37 cases. Ann Pediatr Fenn 1664;10:99-105.

261. Wolff L, Parkinson J, White PD. Bundle branch block with short P-R interval in healthy young people prone to paroxysmal tachycardia. Am Heart J 1930;5:685-704.

262. Liebman J, Plonsey R, Gillette PC. Pediatric electrocardiography. Baltimore: Williams and Wilkins 1982.

263. Michaelsson M, Engle MA. Congenital complete heart block: an international study of the natural history. CV Clinics Brest AN, Engle MA editors. Philadelphia FA Davis 1972.

264. McCue CM, Mantakas ME, Tingstad JB et al Congenital heart block in newborns of mothers with connective tissue disease. Circulation 1977; 56:82-89.

265. Garson A, Gillette PC, McNamara DG. Supraventricular tachycardia in children: clinical features, response to treatment and long term follow up in 217 patients. J Pediatr 1981;98:875-882.

266. Anderson KR, Ho SY, Anderson RH. Location and vascular supply of sinus node in the human heart. Brit Heart J 1979;41:28-32.

267. Gillette P, Reitman M, Gutgesell H et al. Intracardiac electrophysiology in children and young adults. Am Heart J 1975;89:36-44.

268. Sealey WC. The Wolff-Parkinson-White syndrome and the beginnings of direct arrhythmia surgery. Ann Thorac Surg 1984;38:176-180.

269. Kugler JD, Danford DA, Deal BJ, Gillette PC et al. Radiofrequency catheter ablation for tachyarrhythmias in children and adolescents. New Eng J Med 1994;330:1481-1487.

270. Schwartz PJ, Periti M, Malliani A. The long QT syndrome. Am Heart J 1975;89:378-390.

271. Quattlebaum TG, Varghese J, Neill CA, Donahoo JS. Sudden death among postoperative patients with tetralogy of Fallot: a follow-up study of 243 patients for an average of twelve years. Circulation 1976; 54:289-293.

272. Lauer RM, Clarke WR. Use of cholesterol measurements in childhood for the prediction of adult hypercholesterolemia. The Muscatine Study. JAMA 1990;264: 3034-3038.

273. Berenson GS. Cardiovascular risk factors in children. New York, Oxford U Press 1980.

274. Moll PP, Sing CF, Weidman WH, Gordon H, Ellefson RD, Hodgson PA, Kottke BA. Total cholesterol and lipoproteins in school children: prediction of coronary artery disease in adult relatives. Circulation 1983;67:127-134.

275. Kwiterovich PO Jr. Beyond Cholesterol. Baltimore: Johns Hopkins Press, 1989.

276. Bricker JT, Blumenschein SD. Systemic hypertension and preventive cardiology. In: Garson A Jr., Bricker JT, McNamara DG editors. Philadelphia: Lea and Febiger, 1990:1987-1995.

277. Arnesen E, Forsdahl A. The Tromso heart study: Coronary risk factors and their association with living conditions during childhood. J Epidem Comm Health 1985;39:210-214.

278. Report of the second Task Force on blood pressure control in children. Pediatrics 1987;79:1-25.

279. Goldstein JL, Brown MS. The low-density lipoprotein pathway and its relation to atherosclerosis. Ann Rev Biochem 1977;46:897-930.

280. Oliver MF. Dietary fat and coronary heart disease. Brit Heart J 1987;58:423-428.

CHAPTER 7

Development of Pediatric Cardiology

- History of 3 defects, tetralogy, VSD, double inlet ventricle
- Growth of the discipline of pediatric cardiology
- Geographic history

Introduction

We have reviewed in previous chapters some of the sweep of pediatric cardiac advances. Clearly, a number of cardiac defects have extraordinarily fascinating histories, and each defect is separate in the timing of understanding and treatment. Clinically, cardiac problems cannot be thought of in isolation, but always in context of the whole child; but historically, very different tools and concepts were involved in the elucidation of individual defects. An evolutionary approach to the growth of knowledge of 3 specific cardiac anomalies, ventricular septal defect, tetralogy of Fallot, and double inlet ventricle is outlined in the next few pages. Each defect has had its own special problems of recognition and management, and for each new challenges exist in the developmental era.

For ventricular septal defect, many of the questions of prevalence, anatomic variation, and management have been resolved, and the outlook for an infant born with this as an isolated defect is now excellent. Infants with tetralogy of Fallot have also had a dramatic change in the ease, effectiveness and speed of therapy. Many questions remain about the frequency and significance of the extracardiac anomalies so frequently seen with this defect. Double inlet ventricle can now often be successfully treated with modern surgical approaches, but management is still evolving, and etiologic understanding is quite primitive.

The growth of pediatric cardiology as a discipline has been rapid. We will discuss briefly a few of the organisations involved in this growth, including a quotation from Mary Allen Engle, one of the major participants over the past fifty years. Under the heading "geographic cardiology" we will attempt to show how changes and growth have been worldwide, and the geographic diversity of new knowledge and concepts.

Ventricular septal defect

> *"Among the congenital defects of the heart compatible with life and perhaps a long one, one of the most frequent which I have encountered (relatively frequent, absolutely rare) is the communication between the two ventricles because of failure of occlusion of the ventricular septum in its upper portion."*
>
> —Roger H. 1879 quoted in Willius and Keys 1983 [8,51].

Although Roger is rightly best remembered for his graphic description of the murmur and thrill of a ventricular septal defect, he touches in this introductory paragraph on two themes which remained debated for another hundred years, the themes of prevalence and natural history. Defects in the interventricular septum are now generally agreed to be the most common of all congenital cardiac malformations, and to have an extreme range of phenotypic severity. Recent studies in the fetus have confirmed that closure of the septum occurs over a long period in intrauterine life, and likely involves many different genetic mechanisms.

A number of obstacles combined to make the clinical course and natural history of this defect a hotly debated topic until at least late in the 1970's. These obstacles included confusion over the prevalence and type of additional cardiac defects; lack of appreciation of the high rate of associated extracardiac anomalies, some of them severe or life threatening; and a long delay in acceptance of the concept of decreasing size and spontaneous closure of many small defects, particularly those involving the muscular part of the septum.

The history of the ventricular septum started with an error by the great anatomist Galen, living in Pergamon in the second century A.D. In an effort to explain the obvious differences between venous and arterial blood, Galen hypothesised that blood passed between the right and left ventricle through pores in the ventricular septum, pores which he admitted could not be seen. The concept of these "invisible pores" was passed down for centuries, and was not completely abandoned until William Harvey established the true course of the circulation.

It seems probable that now, in the 1990's, we finally have an anatomic understanding of the septum and its defects. The abnormal physiology of the various types of defect is now clear, and corrective surgery, when needed, is available in infancy with extremely low risk. Research continues on details of the embryology of the septum [282], and the pathogenesis of septal defects.

In the three centuries between William Harvey and Maude Abbott much was learned of the possible range of anatomic defects in the ventricular septum. However, physiologic understanding awaited the advent of cardiac catheterisation in the late 1940's, and effective therapy was not available until the 1950's.

During the 100 years separating Roger's paper in 1879 from the publication of the Natural History Study, extraordinary advances had occurred in both physiologic understanding of large and moderate sized defects, and in their treatment. However, successful treatment in infancy, the time of major morbidity and mortality, did not occur till the mid 1970's. The prevalence and natural history of small defects also remained elusive and controversial until the infant era. Not until the last decade, late in the infant era, have the tools of population based epidemiologic study and Doppler echocardiography combined to clarify the story of the small ventricular septal defect.

Table 5
Dates in the History of VSD [2,4,7]

200 AD	Galen's "invisible pores"
1628	Harvey De Motu Cordis
1749	Senac anatomic description of VSD [35]
1782	Hunter anatomic description of VSD in an infant [40]
1879	Roger description of "special cardiac murmur" of VSD [51]
1897	Eisenmenger cyanosis with VSD, "overiding aorta," no PS [69]
1923	Deitlin clinical diagnosis with Xray findings [2]
1936	Abbott statistics, circulatory, auscultatory diagrams [2a]
1952	Muller/Dammann banding of pulmonary artery in infancy [121]
1955	Lillehei [161] Kirklin [164] open repair VSD
1960	Keith [170] spontaneous closure
1970+	Natural History Study [171]
1976	Barratt-Boyes repair in infancy [224]

Rather than reviewing these various contributions sequentially, we will discuss the concepts that were part of the slow evolution of knowledge of this highly variable defect. These concepts include the possibility and refinement of clinical diagnosis, the understanding of pulmonary vascular obstructive disease, the evolution of surgical approaches, and the recognition of spontaneous closure and natural history.

TOOLS AND CONCEPTS IN CLINICAL DIAGNOSIS

It is unclear if anyone had recognised the cardiac murmur as a "pathognomonic sign" prior to Roger's classic description. His complete paper, worth reading in its entirety, is available in translation in Willius and Keyes [8]. One paragraph from Roger's first footnote follows:

> *"In patency of the interventricular septum, I do not see any other cause for the murmur than the flow of blood from left to right across the communication. The mixture of arterial and venous blood which must take place is scarcely contestable, when we recall the differences of pressure which exist, according to the experiments of Marey, between the two ventricles, the force of contraction of the left is equal to 128 millimeters of mercury, that of the right, only 25 ..."*

Henri Roger (1809-1891) was a physician in Paris who had a special interst in both pediatrics and auscultation. Willius and Keys [8] recount that in 1839 Roger and Barth, both then interns, submitted a paper for an award offered by the Societe de Medecine et de Chirurgie de Bordeaux on the role of auscultation; the motto of their paper was: *"If medicine is the most beautiful of the sciences, then auscultation is the most beautiful discovery of modern times."*

In his 1879 paper on ventricular septal defect Roger stated that he had listened to "thousands of children during forty years of special studies." He describes several patients in whom he suspected the presence of a ventricular septal defect because of the long loud systolic murmur and thrill at the left sternal border. These patients had no cyanosis and he comments:

> *"I have concluded with Louis and Gintrac ... that the morbus ceruleus does not arise from the combination of arterial and venous blood, but that it is almost always attributable to a concomitant and likewise congenital lesion, stenosis of the pulmonary artery, the effect of this stenosis being to impede and prevent the arrival of blood in the lungs and consequently the decrease of oxygenation."*

It is interesting that he does not appear to have any concept that pulmonary stenosis might result in increased right ventricular pressure, and thus a right to left shunt. Nevertheless, his discovery shows awareness of the new physiologic data provided by Marey's studies in the normal hearts of laboratory animals [16,55]. Henri Roger's correlation of the long systolic murmur, (later described as "pansystolic" or "holosystolic"), with systolic flow from a high pressure left to a low pressure right ventricle preceded the tool of clinical cardiac catheterisation by 70 years, and the advent of phonocardiography by about 50 years.

Roger mentions the stethoscope several times in his communication, and was clearly familiar with the use of this relatively new tool, originally described by his countryman Rene Theodore Hyacinth Laennec in 1819. In describing his examination of a young man of 17 seeking a certificate of physical fitness for employment as a postman, Roger states:

> *"On applying the ear to the precordial region I heard forthwith a harsh murmur entirely covering the tic-tac of the heart ... and coincidentally a great purring thrill."*

The young man was told he "appeared very capable of carrying out the laborious work of postman." This description is of interest, both in documenting that the role of physicians in signing certificates preceded the 20th century, and also in suggesting that Roger used both direct and indirect methods of auscultation.

In 1861 Roger had described the cardiac findings at necropsy in a twelve year old boy who had died as a result of a comminuted fracture:

> *"... a malformation of the heart which consisted of failure of occlusion of the interventricular septum in its upper portion, without concomitant stenosis of the pulmonary artery ... It goes without saying that this malformation had been completely unrecognised by an entirely pardonable omission on a surgical service, a failure to listen to the heart."*

Roger seems not to have been immune to the common fault of baiting his surgical colleagues. Some of his contemporaries had criticised his original paper because "my clinical description was not based upon a sufficient number of autopsies." It is indeed true, despite the brilliant logic of his arguments, that he lacked autopsy confirmation of his diagnoses. In a later brief communication [8] he describes an acyanotic little girl with an intense systolic murmur and thrill all over the precordium, who died at twenty eight months with autopsy findings of an uncomplicated ventricular septal defect and closed foramen ovale. "This observation gives me proof on all points."

Auscultation and palpation were the only tools of diagnosis directly available to Roger in the latter part of the 19th century. Perhaps the greatest interest in his description lies in his correlation of what he heard with the new information on intracardiac pressures now being gleaned in the experimental physiology laboratory. Like other great men, he was many decades ahead of his time, for the era of clinicophysiologic correlation did not begin in earnest until 70 years later.

The concept that auscultation could sometimes result in a definitive cardiac diagnosis was of course not original to Roger. Peacock had already described the characteristic radiation of the murmur of pulmonic stenosis in 1858, and the location and transmission of the murmur of aortic stenosis was known to Roger, and described in his differential diagnosis.

Other tools of diagnosis had begun to be included by the time of publication of Maude Abbott's Atlas in 1936 [2]. Abbott shows an auscultatory diagram of a characteristic murmur, and gives acknowledgements to Dr Harold Segall, a famous cardiologist of Montreal, for its inclusion. Abbott also reproduces the radiologic findings of cardiomegaly, biventricular enlargement and dilated pulmonary artery described by Dietlin in 1923 [2].

Although Abbott illustrates both a small and a large ventricular septal defect, sophisticated clinical diagnosis of the size of an individual defect, and the correlation of the volume of the left to right shunt with the anatomic size, had to await the tools of both phonocardiography and cardiac catheterisation. (In fact, the development of high quality selective left ventriculography to demonstrate ventricular defect size only briefly preceded the surgeon's direct observation at open repair). Recognition of the importance of an apical mid- diastolic flow rumble, changes in the second heart sound, and the characteristic decrescendo systolic murmur of a small defect in the muscular part of the ventricular septum were all delayed until the late 1950's and early 1960's.

An interesting sub-history could be written on the ups and downs of auscultation during the growth of pediatric cardiology. The discipline owed a great deal to Aubrey Leatham and other cardiologists working mainly with adults, who clarified murmurs by a combination of auscultatory skill and phonocardiography. Extensive studies were needed before the clinical diagnosis of ventricular septal defect was generally agreed, and the clinicophysiologic profile established. The tools of Xray and electrocardiogram were helpful in classifying defects into mild, moderate, severe and inoperable [171], but no single tool dominated until the advent of Doppler echocardiography.

Echocardiography, when first introduced, had impact chiefly on differential diagnosis, since the defect itself could not be visualised by M-mode studies. Although M-mode echocardiography was helpful in differentiating tetralogy from isolated ventricular septal defect, and in some other diagnostic dilemmas, it was not until color Doppler echocardiography became generally available in the mid 1980's that it became possible to clarify the diagnostic spectrum of what Roger described as "failure of occlusion of the interventricular septum."

It had long been suspected that small defects in the muscular septum were frequent, but there was previously no gold standard with which to confirm the diagnosis. Now tiny defects could be confirmed, and later spontaneous closure of such defects established. This new tool also played an extremely important role in excluding additional anomalies, in assessing the rare occasions when cardiac catheterisation might still be needed, and in documenting an intact septum after open repair.

THE CONCEPT OF PULMONARY VASCULAR OBSTRUCTIVE DISEASE

Maude Abbott coined the term "Eisenmenger complex," remarking [2]:

> *"This term has been used by the author, in default of a better, to designate an unusual combination ... of ventricular septal defect with dextroposition of the aorta without any pulmonary stenosis or hypoplasia."*

It would be difficult to think of a term which caused more long term disputation among pediatric cardiologists and others interested in the physiology of the circulation. The problem was, this was a useful shorthand phrase, but the longhand concept it represented was still unknown. The pulmonary vascular bed was still foreign territory. Eventually, by the mid 1970's the term became useful, once pulmonary vascular resistance and pulmonary vascular obstructive disease had reached at least our present interim phase of understanding. What had Eisenmenger actually described? Exactly what Abbott stated.

Eisenmenger in 1897 had described the heart of a young man dying with heart failure and mild cyanosis [69]. Autopsy revealed a large ventricular septal defect and over-riding aorta. Eisenmenger's account is somewhat heavy reading, very different from the lively Roger: indeed it should not be embarked on by anyone making their first dive into historic papers. His communication contains no real suggestion of possible physiology. Interestingly, Abbott reproduces in her Atlas a chest Xray from another patient with this diagnosis dying at 21 years of a brain abscess. The Xray shows not only a dilated main pulmonary artery, but also the classic "pruning" of the pulmonary vessels leaving the hilum, a sign not recognised till two decades later.

Prior to 1940 the concept of pulmonary vascular obstructive disease had not developed. Indeed Abbott includes all defects with intracardiac communications as either in her Group II (cases of arterial venous shunt with terminal reversal of flow (cyanose tardive) or in Group III, with permanent cyanosis. It took many years before the error of the concept was fully recognised, namely that all patients with left to right shunts, no matter how small, might eventually develop reversed flow and cyanosis. The differentiation of ventricular septal defects into restrictive and non-restrictive awaited the 1970's.

Fluoroscopy and chest Xray. By the mid 1940's Taussig had used the tool of the fluoroscope to separate cyanotic patients into two major groups: the first, with pulmonary stenosis and decreased pulmonary vascular markings, (predominantly tetralogy of Fallot), might be helped by an "artificial ductus" or Blalock Taussig shunt. The second, smaller group, with dilated pulsating hilar vessels, often referred to as a "hilar dance" were not candidates for shunt operations.

Cardiac catheterisation shortly thereafter became available to assist in differentiating the larger group of cyanotic patients who might be helped by a shunt, from the much smaller group without pulmonic stenosis. Bing and his associates [283] showed in the catheterisation laboratory that some patients with cyanosis had systemic levels of pulmonary hypertension, and elevated pulmonary vascular resistance.

The pulmonary vascular bed. During the 1950s and 60's attention turned to the microscopy of the pulmonary vascular bed in patients with left to right shunts and other cardiac defects. Jesse Edwards of the Mayo Clinic developed a grading system of the severity of medial hypertrophy and intimal change in the arterioles.

Correlative studies. Physiologic studies in newborn animals and infants defined the normal neonatal changes in pulmonary pressure and resistance levels. While these discoveries were being made, the clinical findings of pulmonary hypertension and increased pulmonary vascular resistance were slowly unfolding. Many contributions came from cardiologists seeing adult patients, who stressed the importance of the pulmonary component of the second heart sound, clinical and electrocardiographic evidence of right ventricular hypertrophy, and the radiologic signs characteristic of pulmonary hypertension. Paul Wood added clarification by emphasising the term "Eisenmenger syndrome," meaning that shunt reversal could occur with a large non restrictive arteriovenous communication at any level, atrial, atrioventricular, ventricular or ductal.

Pulmonary artery banding. Once the concept of pulmonary vascular obstructive disease was recognised, Dammann and Muller [121] pioneered in attempting to halt or reverse what was now shown to be a progressive and ultimately fatal condition. Banding of the pulmonary artery for ventricular or atrioventricular septal defects or double inlet ventricle was life saving in many infants, and allowed them to survive into the era of open repair. The procedure had significant technical difficulties, and some unexpected complications, including acceleration of left ventricular outflow obstruction, but conceptually it was of enormous value in focussing attention on the salvage of the pulmonary vascular bed.

Frank Dammann had a background in physiology and had also worked with Stanley Gibson in Chicago. He joined Helen Taussig as her senior Fellow and first assistant in 1949. In 1951 he left Johns Hopkins to go to UCLA with Harry Muller, one of Dr Blalock's early surgical residents. We are indebted to him for the following unexpurgated notes:

> *"Two special small groups of patients came to my attention and really intrigued the hell out of me while T. was away on her sabbatical; the 'atypical' ductus without a continuous murmur and the 'reverse' ductus. Without exception all of the ducti were large, not small. I do not, and did not believe, as I think T did, that the PVD was an associated defect. I have always thought it was cause and effect, a high pressure high flow because of a very large ductus leading to vascular hypertrophy and then injury. In almost all there was a history of early infant cardiac failure. I wrote up the first group with Gordon Sell and the second with Berthrong ...*
>
> *So I began to look at lung microscopies and soon began to see it as a whole spectrum from congestive failure with normal arteries through clear alveoli with thick walled muscular small pulmonary arteries to the plexiform lesions and totally obstructed arteries of the 'reverse' ductus ...*
>
> *At about the same time Jesse Edwards began writing about Congenital Heart Disease and the lungs. In one of his early (I think) articles, he discussed the case of a man with a single ventricle and transposition without pulmonic stenosis, who had been a hard working farmer and was considered normal until he developed cancer, from which he died. His lungs were normal. On reviewing the heart, Jesse found a ledge of tissue under the pulmonary valve which he thought just enough to cut his pulmonary resting blood flow to perhaps twice systemic, enough to permit normal exercise without visible cyanosis in an outdoor type individual. Says I to myself, "Why not do the same to these babies? Let's reduce the size of the pulmonary artery electively." I felt sure that we could do two things; correct the extreme high output failure that these babies had, and stop and probably reverse the hypertrophic muscular changes occurring in the small pulmonary arteries and arterioles ... I remember talking to Al Blalock and suggesting banding the pulmonary artery, but I dont remember what we decided to do about it. I think I was too close to moving West ...*

Dammann describes how Dr Blalock did attempt banding in one infant with a truncus arteriosus, sent to surgery with the erroneous diagnosis of atypical patent ductus. The infant did not survive. Dammann and Muller then moved to UCLA, and continued to work intensively on the experimental production of large left to right shunts in the laboratory, on techniques of banding and on the study of the pulmonary vascular bed in lung biopsies and at pathology.

> *"From the dog lab we went to the OR. The first baby was six months of age, with an AV canal, one pound over birth weight and all of that edema fluid ... The Tiger, as he was known at the hospital, had a rough time for a couple of days, but then did very well for some 8 or ten years, until another team tried to correct his canal, could not and lost him."*
>
> —J. Francis Dammann M.D. Professor emeritus of cardiology University of Virginia Charlottesville VA. Quoted with permission.

This brief communication reminds us of the stormy passage of many children, families and physicians as heart surgery was evolving. This infant had pioneered as pulmonary artery banding developed, and again when undergoing open heart surgery in 1964. This was only a few years before Rastelli's classic paper in 1968 [182], which described the optimal technique for repairing atrioventricular septal defects, and thereby vastly improved postoperative mortality and morbidity.

Historically, the majority of infants who underwent successful banding of the pulmonary artery had ventricular septal defects. Banding also came to be used experimentally in the study of progression and regression of myocardial hypertrophy, and in many embryologic studies.

Pulmonary Vascular Obstructive Disease in the Infant era. Work from a number of centers, primarily the Mayo Clinic, had made it clear during the early 1970s that reversal of pulmonary vascular disease was unlikely to occur if closure of a ventricular or atrioventricular septal defect was delayed past infancy. Since the advent of the infant surgical era, pulmonary vascular disease is rarely if ever seen, since infants at risk can and do have corrective surgery in the first few months of life.

Attempts to treat pulmonary vascular disease, particularly primary pulmonary hypertension, with medications, were slow and intensely frustrating. Only now, with the use of calcium channel blockers and occasionally of continuous prostacyclin infusions in the home, is some progress being made. Increasingly sophisticated techniques are now available to study the pulmonary vascular bed.

CONCEPT OF DIMINUTION IN SIZE OR SPONTANEOUS CLOSURE OF VSD

Roger had emphasised the benign prognosis of ventricular septal defect in many patients, but shortly after the advent of the therapeutic era attention shifted to the defect as a frequent cause of congestive heart failure, early infant death or delayed pulmonary vascular disease. Some authoritative, if pessimistic, cardiologists believed that the comparative rarity of ventricular septal defects in adults was entirely due to premature deaths. When Evans, Rowe and Keith described in 1960 the spontaneous closure of some defects [170], they met with a sceptical reception. French [284] had written, some 42 years earlier:

> *"Some years ago I saw a small boy, 14 months old, and on examination ... there was a very loud systolic bruit, with its maximum intensity over the fourth intercostal space, close to the sternum ... accompanied by a thrill ... the diagnosis made by myself and others was congenital perforation of the interventricular septum. The father of the boy was in the Navy ... and it was a tremendous blow to him to find that the child had a bruit which was certain to cause his rejection at the medical examination ... In my ignorance, I gave the opinion that it was useless to think of the boy's some day being eligible for the Navy or indeed for any service in which a physical examination had to be passed. Most clinicians would, I think, have given the same opinion as I did; but it was wrong; and that is why I want you to know about it. I saw the boy again when he was two years old, and the bruit was about the same ... I saw him again when he was five and there was then absolutely no bruit at all! The father's keen desire that the boy should follow him in the service has since been gratified and the case has taught me that the bruit of a congenital malformation of the heart may disappear as the child grows up."*

This highly "anecdotal," gratifyingly succinct account is interesting in suggesting that in 1918, about 39 years after Roger's report, the specificity of the cardiac murmur of ventricular septal defect was widely accepted. It is also an enjoyable reminder that in the past, a few cardiologists did not claim infallibility as a natural right.

During the 1950's the use of cardiac catheterisation as the gold standard for diagnosis resulted in underestimation of the prevalence of small ventricular septal defects. Even the most enthusiastic proponents of cardiac catheterisation were seldom willing to undertake the procedure in a child with a loud murmur but absolutely no clinical, radiographic or electrocardiographic sign of any physiologic disturbance.

By 1970 the Natural History and other studies had clearly documented by left ventriculography that spontaneous closure or diminution in size of ventricular defects could occur. Another period of disagreement ensued as to the source of the billowing tissue seen restricting some small, or even previously large, defects, and decreasing shunt size. Use of the unfortunate term "aneurysm of the ventricular septum" did not finally prevent consensus that the occluding tissue was almost invariably derived from the tricuspid valve. Twenty seven years after Evans, and 60 years after French, Moe and Gunteroth [285] used Doppler echocardiography in an interesting way to answer the deceptively simple question "How many defects undergo spontaneous closure?" The answer, as is often the case with simple sounding questions, was "It all depends on the population studied." In their study, of 44 infants with a ventricular septal defect followed from birth, 20 (45%) underwent spontaneous closure by one year of age. By contrast, among 165 infants referred from outside for evaluation, spontaneous closure occurred in 37 (22%). Surgical closure was required in 30/165 referred defects. Their study, unlike some others, did not show significant differences in closure rates depending on the site or size of the defect.

The tool of the Doppler echocardiogram has also been of tremendous value in documenting tiny or multiple ventricular defects which could previously be diagnosed on ausculation but not confirmed by other methods.

CONCEPTS OF PREVALENCE AND NATURAL HISTORY

It took almost 100 years before Roger's generalisation regarding ventricular septal defect, that it was "relatively frequent, absolutely rare," was accompanied by hard figures. One great difficulty in assessing prevalence was the frequent combination of ventricular septal defect with other cardiac anomalies. This difficulty was gradually overcome with the growth of hierarchical classification systems, so that each patient received only one primary anatomic diagnosis. One of the many enduring contributions of the New England Regional Infant Cardiac Program lay in the use of such a hierarchical approach, so that an infant with a ventricular septal defect and patent ductus would be classified as having a septal defect; one with a coarctation and ventricular septal defect as having a coarctatation.

True prevalence data also had to await population based studies, the definition of prevalence at live birth, and the advent of color Doppler technology for the confirmation of the presence of small ventricular septal defects in infancy. Martin and his colleagues did a valuable study showing the interaction of technology and prevalence data [286]. The use of color Doppler technology caused an apparent rise in the prevalence of small ventricular septal defects, particularly those involving the muscular septum; the prevalence of defects needing repair in infancy, or accompanied by extracardiac anomalies, has shown little change [217]. Henri Roger did not forsee the complexity of scientific precision.

Consensus on the management of ventricular septal defect is approaching, if not yet complete. Some would advocate closure of even small defects if they have not closed by late childhood, citing the low surgical risk and the avoidance of future endocarditis. Others feel that echocardiography is so sensitive in diagnosing which defects will ultimately get smaller, that surgery in infancy can be delayed in an infant with a defect less than half the size of the aortic root, who is showing signs of persistent mild heart failure and poor growth. Between these poles of surgical eagerness and medical domination by new technology, a path will be found. The prognosis for a child born with a large ventricular septal defect has improved vastly since Roger examined his aspiring postman [287]. It is likely that future cardiologists will be fortunate enough never to see an infant die due to a ventricular septal defect, and never encounter Eisenmenger syndrome in an adult.

Tetralogy of Fallot

The chronicle of tetralogy of Fallot is part of a dramatic evolution in cardiology, cardiac surgery, and understanding of the developing heart [288]. Many new tools and concepts have evolved in the three hundred years since Steno of Denmark first described the defect in 1673, and particularly in the century since Fallot of Marseilles coined the term tetralogy in 1888. By the time of the culmination of the first era, that of pathologic anatomy, in 1936, Maude Abbott was able to include in her Atlas some information on clinical findings in addition to pathology [2].

The therapeutic age began with the first Blalock Taussig anastomosis in 1944, followed by open heart repair 10 years later. The third, or infant era, beginning in the mid 1970's, brought many advances for an infant born with tetralogy of Fallot. These advances included the possibility of successful primary intracardiac repair in infancy, the use of echocardiography for early and precise noninvasive diagnosis, and the introduction of prostaglandin therapy. The 4th current era of cardiac development, beginning in the 1990's, gives hope for early understanding of the molecular basis of tetralogy

THE ERA OF PATHOLOGIC ANATOMY

In 1673 Steno, also known as Nils Stensen, gave what is possibly the earliest account of this cardiac malformation [36,37]. His description, followed by many others in the age of pathologic anatomy, began to lay the foundation for the first Blalock Taussig shunt in 1944.

Steno described the findings in a stillborn infant who had a bifid sternum and omphalocele in addition to tetralogy, a combination sometimes now termed Pentalogy of Cantrell. The infant also had syndactyly, and "a cleft palate and hare-lip on the right side, and the mother attributed this anomaly to the fact that she was fond of rabbit stew." Steno reproduces her teratologic theory without comment, but says of the cardiac abnormality "As to the cause of this phenomenon, I have nothing to say." While applauding Steno's admirable reticence, his story suggests that parental concern as to the cause of malformations was as intense then as it remains today, and is also a salutary reminder that extracardiac defects are important and frequent in tetralogy of Fallot [289]. It was to be approximately 200 years until the beginnings of teratology as a science, and 300 years until Ferencz [217] embarked on the systematic search for risk factors for congenital heart defects. Further case reports followed, and in 1784 William Hunter [40] gave a graphic description of cyanotic spells:

> *"The most distressing symptoms were fits, which were always alarming ... When the fit was coming upon him, he was commonly sensible of it; he grew oppressed at his heart, became weak or faint, grew dark in his colour, and at last almost black, fell down and seemed insensible. He commonly soon came out of the fit, with sobbing and yawning, and a sense of fatigue..."* Later, commenting on the growth pattern: *"His figure was very extraordinary. In height, he was nearly what might be expected at his age: but he was not much in thickness in any part of his body. And though he was remarkably thin, he had not the look of being wasted by consumption; on the contrary, it appeared to be his natural habit. If a man had never seen any of the canine species but the bulldog, for example, he would be much struck at the first sight of the slender and delicate Italian greyhound"* ... and later in the text *"why there was not the full effect of nutrition, or why he did not increase in thickness as well as in length, I leave to be explained by those philosophers who know exactly the whole process of nutrition ..."*

Peacock in the 1850's, had noted the characteristic radiation of the murmur of pulmonary stenosis, and by the time Fallot wrote in 1888, there were many clinical and pathologic reports available for his review. Fallot's analysis led him to destroy the prevailing concept that cardiac cyanosis was always due to patency of the foramen ovale. All subsequent workers are indebted to him for this advance, his recognition that this was the most common of all cyanotic defects, and his use of the liberating term "tetralogie." Fallot's review includes a surprisingly large number of adults, perhaps because autopsies in young infants were rarely performed, and even more rarely reported, in an era of high infant mortality.

By 1936 Maude Abbott was able to illustrate circulatory and auscultatory diagrams, the chest Xray and 3 lead electrocardiogram in tetralogy. It was probably her use of the term tetralogy of Fallot that assured its acceptance into the world of famous and enduring eponyms. Although Maude Abbott was not a clinician, she was greatly interested in the correlation of clinical and pathologic findings, the emerging concept of a specific clinical profile for each defect. Table 1 summarises a few important dates in the understanding of tetralogy of Fallot. Any table of major contributions is unsatisfactory and incomplete. This particular table is intended to emphasise the theme that pediatric cardiology has progressed from anatomic studies to physiology, therapy, and now an intense interest in etiology and pathogenesis.

Table 6
Dates in the history of tetralogy of Fallot [2,4,7,288]

■ 1628	Harvey normal circulation
■ 1673	Steno tetralogy
■ 1777	Sandifort tetralogy
■ 1784	Hunter cyanotic spells
■ 1819	Laennec stethoscope
■ 1847	Chevers tetralogy with absent pulmonary valve
■ 1858	Peacock localisation of murmur
■ 1870	Fick principle
■ 1888	Fallot cyanosis in "tetralogie"
■ 1936	Abbott clinicopathologic profile
■ 1944	Blalock Taussig shunt
■ 1946	Catheterisation angiography
■ 1955	Open repair Lillehei, Kirklin
■ 1975	Primary repair in infancy Barratt Boyes, Castaneda
■ 1976	Prostaglandin therapy Olley
■ 1970+	Di George, Shprintzen syndromes
■ 1980	neural crest involvement RV outflow

When Steno wrote his original description, no concept of possible future therapy seems to have occurred to him, nor indeed to legions of subequent writers. The table above illustrates two themes, the tools and concepts of therapy, and the theme of pathogenesis, or "why did it happen?" the theme voiced by the mother in Steno's report, and by countless parents since.

THE CONCEPT OF THERAPY

Some account has already been given in chapter 4 of the history of the early Blalock Taussig shunt procedure. The effect of the operation was electrifying, and it gained world wide acceptance. In 1947, Blalock and Taussig gave a combined lecture in the great hall of the British Medical Association in London. Brock, as quoted by Mark Ravitch [86], described the culmination of the lecture in the now darkened hall: a spotlight shone on:

> *"a small cherublike girl of 2½ years with a halo of blond curly hair and looking pink and well; she had been operated on at Guy's by Blalock a week earlier ... no one there could possibly forget it."*

That dramatic moment symbolised that pediatric cardiology and cardiac surgery were now inextricably linked, and were international. The surgery was indeed only palliative, but the curse of "incurability" had been lifted from tetralogy of Fallot.

The advent of cardiopulmonary bypass and open repair of tetralogy in the mid 1950's signalled a remarkable advance, one ultimately leading to the present era of primary repair in infancy. However, the decade of the late 1950's and early 1960's was in some ways a difficult time for patients, families and physicians, since the mortality of open repair remained high for some years.

It was a time when many patients underwent one or more shunt procedures prior to open repair [290]. There was controversy over whether prior shunt procedures increased the risk. It became apparent that previous direct aorto-pulmonary anastomoses greatly increased the hazards of intracardiac surgery, while Blalock Taussig anastomoses did not. Anastomoses between the subclavian and pulmonary artery tended to grow smaller over the years, due to fibrosis at the anastomotic site; thus, over a period ranging between five and fifteen years, nearly all patients had a recurrence of cyanosis and polycythemia and required further intervention. By contrast, many aortopulmonary shunts grew larger, and although the patient might be almost free of cyanosis and polycythemia, major complications occurred at subsequent open repair due to pulmonary artery distortion and often associated pulmonary hypertension.

Cardiologists, surgeons and pathologists collaborated in long term follow up studies. Late postoperative arrhythmias were a particular subject of concern. These seem less of a problem now, probably due to a combination of improved myocardial protection, and earlier age at repair.

Anatomic Variations had been recognised as occurring in tetralogy, and the clinical profile was known to be more severe in those with pulmonary outflow atresia rather than stenosis. Variations became of much greater import once the heart was to be surgically opened. There was increasing recognition of the need for anatomic precision, a need reviewed from a surgical viewpoint by Kirklin and Karp in their monograph of 1970 [291], and in a number of studies of pathologic anatomy. During the two decades between the advent of cardiopulmonary bypass and the beginning of the infant era, much attention was paid to the extraordinary degree of anatomic variation which could occur, and new surgical approaches were devised. In 1988 both Robert Anderson and Richard van Praagh attended the meeting in Marseilles honoring the centenary of Fallot's original publication. They each reviewed Fallot's contribution, and described the new anatomic and pathologic concepts which had been added in the past 100 years [72,73].

In the Infant Era beginning in the mid 1970's, three major changes profoundly affected patients with tetralogy of Fallot: the introduction of prostaglandins, advances in infant surgery, and the rise of echocardiography. Invasive cardiology played a much smaller role.

The successful medical manipulation of the ductus was of tremendous benefit to many neonates, including the approximately 20% of all infants with tetralogy born with pulmonary outflow atresia. It was not until the mid 1980's that primary repair of tetralogy of Fallot in infancy became the norm, as surgeons around the world followed the pioneering lead of Barratt-Boyes and Castaneda [224,225].

Echocardiography was of great benefit in allowing for early and accurate diagnosis; of historic interest was the ability to visualise immediately, even on M-Mode echocardiography, that most elusive of the components of Fallot's tetrad, the aortic over-ride. Cardiac catheterisation began to be used only for immediate preoperative assessment, and there is increasing likelihood that most infants with tetralogy will be able to have open repair without any prior invasive procedures.

The graphic phrase "And it happened in our lifetime" [292], was used by Dr Vincent Gott as the title of his paper on how therapy for tetralogy of Fallot, a relatively rare disorder, was followed so rapidly by the ongoing revolution in cardiovascular therapy. Vince Gott was a resident with Lillehei in Minneapolis during the first open heart operations, and later succeeded Alfred Blalock as chief of cardiovascular surgery at Johns Hopkins. Dr William Glenn, another highly innovative surgeon, conveyed the same idea; demonstrating his exhibit on heart surgery at Yale University [88] with his long time colleague, Dr Ruth Whittemore, on an icebound New England winter day in 1994, he exclaimed: "Weren't we lucky to have been alive then, and part of it?"

WHY DID IT HAPPEN?

Progress in studies of pathogenesis has been significant, if less widely known. During the 270 years from Steno to the dawn of the therapeutic age major contributions were made to embryology and theories of pathogenesis, many reviewed by Abbott [2], and later by van Mierop [61].

The concept that tetralogy was due to abnormal partitioning of the primitive conotruncus was generally accepted by the middle of this century, but teratologic studies had not proven fruitful, and epidemiologic analyses were not yet available. The tragic episode of thalidomide embryopathy in the 1960's [137,138] gave a new urgent impetus to teratologic research. New methods of labelling cells migrating into primitive right ventricular outflow tract led to recognition of the crucial role of neural crest cells in conotruncal development [211,212].

Almost simultaneously, during the mid 1970's, two major contributions were made to the recognition of clinical syndromes associated with tetralogy of Fallot. During the early years of therapy, extracardiac malformations had received relatively little attention, probably because shunt operations were difficult in infancy, and were mostly undertaken only if other major defects were absent. The mortality of a cyanotic infant with another severe defect such as cleft palate was very high. The velofaciocardiac syndrome was described by Shprintzen in a series of papers starting in the mid 1970's [293]. In 1972 Freedom and associates drew attention to cardiac anomalies, including severe tetralogy of Fallot, in Di George syndrome [294]. Many subsequent reports have followed, and with the use of new microbiologic techniques it now seems probable tetralogy is one component of a multiple organ system defect linked to a deletion of the TUPLE 1 gene on the long arm of chromosome 22.

How many patients with tetralogy have what is catchingly called the CATCH22 syndrome is not yet certain, but it is very reasonable to speculate that the infant described by Steno was one of them. Clearly genetic factors are at the intersection of the clinical spectrum and the biology of tetralogy of Fallot. Studies in animal models, and family and epidemiologic studies, have all contributed to an increased understanding of this phenotypically varied defect, known to medicine for the past 300 years.

Double Inlet Ventricle

Several issues arise in discussing the history of this complex group of defects. Nomenclature has been a persisting difficulty; the term cor triloculare biatrium, (meaning a three chambered heart with two atria), was widely used in the 18th and 19th century. In retrospect, this term had certain advantages; it was universally understood, it avoided a specific statement that there was only a "single" ventricle, (when in fact there were almost always 2 ventricular cavities of markedly unequal size), and it ignored argument over the embryologic origin of the large ventricle. Also, by sheer sonority of phrasing, it conveyed the fact that this was a difficult, possibly heterogeneous, and challenging problem. With the demise of Latin as a common language, many controversies arose over nomenclature, which are only now yielding to consensus.

THE ERA OF PATHOLOGIC ANATOMY

According to Rashkind [7], there were several anatomic descriptions of this defect in the 17th and 18th century, from that of Pozzis in 1676 to Mery in 1700. The report by Holmes in 1824 [295] was thus far from the first to describe double inlet ventricle. His communication is of historic interest for several reasons. The heart specimen was preserved, and must have travelled with Holmes when he emigrated from Edinburgh to Montreal. Safely ensconsed in the McGill Museum, the "unique" case

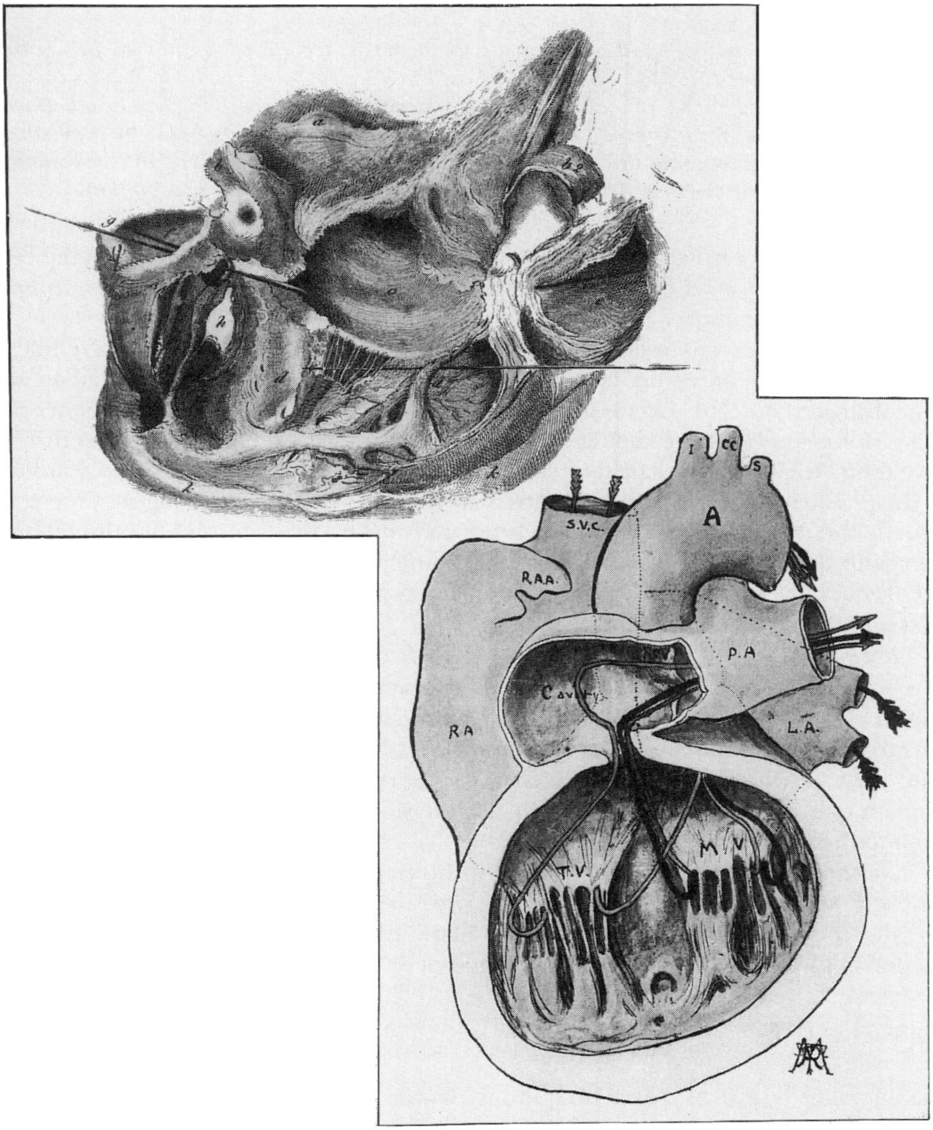

PLATE III.
Diagrammatic sketch by Dr. R. Tait Mackenzie, showing course of blood and relation of cavities. The pale line shows venous blood, the dark line arterial blood,

Figure 15—The Holmes Heart The original drawing by Holmes was reproduced by Abbott in 1901, and she added the circulatory diagram.

attracted the attention of Osler, who maintained that he taught on it and encouraged Maude Abbott to redescribe it in detail [17]. She did so in one of her earliest papers [296], and she was so intrigued by the findings that her determination to make cardiac defects her life work was reinforced, and the scientific categorisation of defects began. Holmes wrote:

> *"The following case of malformation of the heart is, I believe, unique, so far as the appearances extend ... Many of the cases collected by Dr Farre resemble this in one or more particulars, but no one exactly ... the patient was a 22 year old man of a delicate habit, ... affected from infancy with a palpitation of the heart, attended by a peculiar blueness of the cheeks and lips ... The oedema increased gradually ... and in consequence of enlargement of the liver being perceived, submuriate of mercury was conjoined."*

In describing the cardiac anatomy, Holmes states that the large ventricle is the left ventricle, and the small chamber *"the remaining part of the right ventricle. To this portion the pulmonary artery remains attached."*

Abbott, in her comments 80 years later, remarks on Holmes careful clinical observations, but notes his lack of reference to either percussion, described by Augenbrugger in 1761, or to stethoscopic auscultation, attributed to Laennec in 1819. Holmes, even if he indulged in a stethoscope, may well, like his successors, have found the techniques of ausculatation and percussion disturbingly unrewarding in this anomaly. He may have preferred to remain silent on the enigma they presented. The patient may have had no heart murmur in early life, and developed one later with the onset of cardiac failure and insufficiency of the atrioventricular valve. This sequence, now well recognised, remained puzzling to most clinicians for at least another one hundred and fifty years.

Abbott added 3 illustrations to the original copper engraving in Holmes' paper. It is interesting to compare the original engraving with her circulatory diagram (Figure 15). Abbott, in commenting that her diagram *"shows the mixed course of the blood and the relation of its cavities. It will be seen that no chamber contains pure arterial blood,"* has thus added the concept of intracardiac mixing. In her diagram she is seeking to show both the physiology and anatomy of the famous "Holmes heart."

Neither Abbott nor Holmes allude to the fact that in this form of double inlet ventricle, without pulmonic stenosis, the pressure in the pulmonary artery must at all times be equal to systemic pressure. Many new tools and concepts would be needed before classification, clinical diagnosis or therapy could begin.

CLASSIFICATION

Classification is a dreaded, if ubiquitous, word. Anderson and Becker, who have contributed so much to new knowledge of anatomopathology in the 20th century, open a recent chapter on the anatomy and pathology of valvular stenosis [177a] with a section "definition of terms." They remark that, to some readers, "definition" has the same effect as has "culture" on the man whose reaction was to release the safety catch of his Browning revolver. (Wenn ich Kultur hore ... entsichere ich meinen Browning" from the play Schlageter by Hanns Johst) ... In the hazardous modern cities of Los Angeles or Baltimore, the weapon drawn in response to terms such as definition or classification might well be an automatic repeater rifle.

Nevertheless, it seems to have been in Baltimore that the first attempts to classify this highly contentious defect were made. By 1947 Taussig had recognised that some forms of "single ventricle" were associated with pulmonic stenosis, and that cyanotic patients might be helped by a shunt operation. Thus, in a sense, therapy preceded both a precise clinical diagnosis and a generally accepted classification. Taussig also taught that the response to a shunt procedure and the long term outcome was less predictable and satisfactory than in tetralogy of Fallot. She described how the rudimentary outlet chamber might be either subaortic or subpulmonary, and the arteries as either normally related or transposed.

All recent classifications have built on the pioneering work of Richard van Praagh, and his wife and colleague Stella, who met on a collaborative study of dextrocardia while one was working in Toronto, the other in Buffalo. Both had at different times been Fellows in pediatric cardiology with Helen Taussig, and remained her close friends during their later distinguished careers in Boston. Maurice Lev had already begun to classify complex heart defects, but Van Praagh's introduction of the "segmental approach" in 1964 was critical to understanding of the double inlet heart. The concept that the atria and visceral situs should be analysed separately from the ventricles and great arteries, and that each chamber had a distinctive morphology, brought order to a cacophony of nomenclature [297]. He also coined the term "situs ambiguus" for the heterotaxy syndromes.

Anderson and his colleagues [298] made great contributions by stressing the primacy of sequence and connections. Although there is not yet a consensus on the optimal terminology, double inlet ventricle can now be internationally classified and defined.

In looking at the Holmes heart (Fig 14) it is true that the large ventricle has the morphologic features we all now know, thanks to our pathologic colleagues, to be characteristic of the left ventricle. Did Holmes, 170 years ago, know that? Did he call the large cavity the "left" ventricle because of its morphology, because it looked to him like other left ventricles in normal hearts; or did he make the "correct" call simply because the chamber lay to the left? He may simply have been fortunate his patient did not have dextrocardia; we will never know for sure.

CLINICAL DIAGNOSIS

Auscultation was not helpful, but Helen Taussig recognised early that the cardiac contour on chest xray and fluoroscopy was usually significantly different in double inlet ventricle from that in tetralogy of Fallot. Partly, this was because the shadow of the ascending aorta frequently made up the left heart border, giving a contour readily separable from the boot shaped heart of tetralogy. By the early 1950's, after precordial leads were available, left axis deviation, or an abnormal superior vector, in a cyanotic patient was shown to be a clue to double inlet ventricle and tricuspid atresia. Much work attempting to correlate the precordial leads with intracardiac anatomy was overall unavailing. A patient with much intracardiac mixing, as in the Holmes heart and other variants, remained a diagnostic dilemma until high quality selective angiocardiography and the new classification were combined by the 1970's.

CONCEPTS OF THERAPY

Although Glenn had introduced the concept of using a venous-pulmonary artery anastomosis to bypass the right side of the heart in 1954 [105], the method was not used systematically on a widespread basis for at least another two decades. Patients with double inlet ventricle underwent a variety of different approaches, partly because of the basic heterogeneity of the defect, and partly because of persisting technical problems with venous bypass methods.

Shunt procedures, usually systemic but sometimes venous, benefited some patients with pulmonic stenosis and double inlet ventricle. Those without pulmonic stenosis who developed signs of congestive heart failure often underwent banding of the pulmonary artery. However, a patient who was not severely symptomatic might not be so treated, and by the time the Fontan procedure became available, a number of unfortunate patients were ineligible, having already developed pulmonary vascular obstructive disease. There were probably two reasons: first, the rationale for preserving the pulmonary vascular bed was less clear in this complex anomaly than in others, in which future definitive repair was already conceptualised: and second, the results of banding tended to be discouraging in this condition for a variety of reasons.

Fontan of Bordeaux reported in 1971 [183] a method of atrial to pulmonary bypass which was a conceptual and technical breakthrough of major proportions for those born without two adequate ventricles. The original results proved better in tricuspid atresia than in double inlet ventricle. The Fontan operation has now a vast literature of its own, describing innumerable modifications. Because the number of patients eligible for the procedure is relatively small worldwide, while the technical difficulties are numerous, one could wish in retrospect that some regionalisation of surgery could have been agreed upon. Other surgical approaches involving ventricular septation proved of benefit to a selected group.

Today, using Doppler echocardiography, it is possible to make an accurate noninvasive diagnosis in a neonate or even a fetus with double inlet ventricle. Modern management concentrates on avoiding distortion of the pulmonary arteries: thus systemic to pulmonary arterial shunts are, if possible, eschewed. Preservation of the pulmonary vascular bed by banding the pulmonary artery is less popular than in the past. If feasible, early performance of a bidirectional Glenn procedure is followed a few months later by completion of the Fontan operation. In infants with a small bulboventricular foramen and levotransposed great arteries, other operations including Damos Kay Stanzel have been proposed.

The vagaries of the history of pediatric cardiology have not yet provided a large cohort of adults of twenty three years or older who have successfully run the gamut of modern approaches to therapy, but the cohort is slowly growing. It might indeed make an excellent collaborative project for cardiologists and surgeons available and interested in the year 2024, to analyse the course and status of all patients worldwide, born with double inlet ventricle, who have outlived the young man described by Holmes 200 years before.

The Growth of Pediatric Cardiology

In 1944 there was no recognised specialty of pediatric cardiology, although a few physicians, including Helen Taussig in Baltimore and Stanley Gibson in Chicago, were known to have a particular interest in heart disease in children. At an update meeting in 1972, almost 30 years later, Blumenthal reported [218] that there were 300 individuals certified as specialists in pediatric cardiology; this number was 884 in 1991 [299], and has now increased to almost 1,000 in the mid 1990's. The growth of the specialty in the United States has been accompanied by similar world wide expansion [300].

Dan McNamara in 1983, a decade after the meeting described by Blumenthal, wrote an original and very readable review of medical advances in the field [176]. McNamara trained with Helen Taussig in the early 1950's, and then went to Houston Texas, where he established his own major and diversified center of pediatric cardiology; Denton Cooley, formerly a resident with Dr Alfred Blalock, was his surgical colleague. McNamara, in writing of medical advances of the quarter century 1958 to 1983, analysed a group of eight major advances, and listed 35 others. His paper remains a valuable source of references and of analytic thinking.

McNamara wrote that advances in medical treatment may give rise to less public acclaim than surgical feats, but that organisational changes and medical developments had also been important in improved patient outcome and in acquisition of new knowledge. He stressed the varied background of such developments, many arising from clinical or laboratory discoveries later applied to pediatrics. Since he began building his own Division in 1952, it is not clear why he chose 1958 as the start of his narrative, except that this choice of dates provided him with a neatly rounded quarter of a century of progress!

Under the heading **developments in the organization of the discipline of pediatric cardiology** he wrote of the establishment of the subspecialty; in January 1958 approximately 30 pediatricians were devoting most or all of their time to heart disease in children.

McNamara described the growth of the Sub-Board of pediatric cardiology of the American Academy of Pediatrics. The Sub-Board's original members were James W. DuShane of the Mayo Clinic, Forrest H. Adams of UCLA, Edward C. Lambert of Buffalo, Alexander S. Nadas of Boston, Saul J. Robinson of San Francisco and Helen B. Taussig of Baltimore. As the Sub-Board and its diplomates grew in numbers and influence, an early study of their activities in 1967 revealed that academicians were spending very little time in research; efforts were made to remedy this, but the conflicting claims of patient care and research remain a problem even now, a decade after McNamara wrote.

Other professional societies contributed to growth in stature and influence of the discipline, including the Council on Cardiovascular Disease in the Young of the American Heart Association (formerly the Council on Rheumatic Fever and Congenital Heart Disease), and the committee on pediatric cardiology of the American College of Cardiology. Programs supported by the Federal Government included the Inter-Society Commission for Heart Disease resources, whose report in 1971 set standards used by many centers. The Crippled Children's Services, developed in the 1960s, and research and training grants and grants-in-aid of the National Heart Lung and Blood Institute were other important federal endeavors.

The establishment of fellowship training programs, the development of accepted standards of care, and the attraction of a rapidly growing and exciting body of knowledge, all ensured that a cadre of excellent young physicians began to join the discipline. McNamara comments that program directors began to increase the amount of time fellows and junior faculty could spend in research and investigation. As cardiac knowledge as a whole became more diversified and complex, the best programs fostered some sub-sub-specialisation, with one or more member of the group focussing attention on hemodynamics, arrhythmia studies, or echocardiography, as the importance of each became apparent. McNamara lists the improved diagnosis and management of pediatric arrhythmias as one of the eight major advances since 1958; his own group, including for some years both Paul Gillette and Arthur (Tim) Garson, were major leaders in this field of knowledge.

Advances required skill, interest and ingenuity, but also protected laboratory time; in retrospect it seems clear that new diversified groupings were an essential component of a valuable division. The formation and nurturing of such groups could only occur in a University setting with a large volume of patients, a good and active surgical program, a supportive administration, and a division head with vision of a changing field and a personality allowing for the growth of others. This was not an easy constellation of circumstance and individual achievement, and much credit is due to those who succeeded. No longer the first generation of pioneers, division directors in the quarter century analysed by McNamara were, in a sense, like heirs to a famous dynasty. It was, and is, hard to build, even on great foundations. It was easier to keep on in the old ways of generalism in pediatric cardiology, rather than create new systems. Fortunately, many did succeed.

Mary Allen Engle, has recently shared with us some of her perspectives on the past 50 years:

My Impressions of Pediatric Cardiology as it Grew and Developed.
by Mary Allen Engle M.D., Professor Emeritus of Pediatrics, Stavros S. Niarchos Professor emerita of pediatric cardiology, New York Hospital-Cornell University Medical College New York NY.

"I was lucky to be a fourth year medical student and substitute intern on the Childrens Surgical Service at Hopkins in November and December 1944, when the miracle of the first Blalock Taussig operation occurred. Denton Cooley was the assistant resident, Harry Muller his senior, and Bill Longmire was the chief resident. What an exciting time! No

wonder that we all continued in the fields Drs Blalock and Taussig were beginning to develop.

During my Pediatric residency and assistant residency, Richard Bing started the cardiac catheterisation laboratory and Bob Cooley began to do angiocardiograms, uniplane, with a changer pushed beneath the patient on the table from one side to the other for a series of films.

It was a privilege to become one of Dr Taussig's first fellows. Emphasis then was on handling the vast numbers of patients being referred from all over the world ... Dr Taussig's book was published at just the right time (first edition 1947). It immediately became the bible for all of us interested in this new field.

Without calling it continuing education, as we do now, Dr Taussig began a reunion every two years of her former fellows. It started with a picnic with crabcakes on her lawn. For three days ... current fellows presented new material and follow ups, while former fellows shared their experiences. At the first reunion Alex Nadas and John Keith were invited and adopted into this loyal group ..."

Engle then described writing with Helen Taussig the two major papers which defined the clinical spectrum of pulmonic valvar stenosis and Ebstein anomaly. After going to New York Hospital-Cornell she continued her interest in pulmonic stenosis: analysing the pathology specimens availabe at New York Hospital she realised the importance of severe malformations in infants, and wrote on the recognition and management of heart failure in young babies. From the outset she collaborated with the surgeons, even to working with them in the dog lab, and she later made a series of contributions on postpericardiotomy syndrome. Her letter continues:

"In 1954 committee work began for me. In the American Academy of Pediatrics, that committe, ably chaired by Jim DuShane, resulted in the establishment of the first subspecialty section (the Section on Cardiology) and the first subspecialty boards that the Academy permitted. In the American Heart Association ... we began a series of meetings with medical officers of insurance companies to improve the status of people with congenital heart disease, unoperated or postoperative, in regard to their insurability and employability. This led to efforts by a number of us that are still not wholly successful: to insure compassionate, informed care long term for adults with congenital heart disease ...

In New York City and then in New York State, the Cardiac Advisory Committee established and enforced guidelines for care ... and we began to collect statistics that documented the steady decline in mortality rates ...

I did nothing to develop echocardiography, but I applaud the enormous benefits derived. Each individual with congenital heart disease, from the fetus to the elderly, can potentially benefit from this technique. Invasive, therapeutic cardiology has already proven its worth in my original favorite condition, pulmonic stenosis, and in time it appears likely that the problems with other lesions..will be worked out. In 1980 Kawasaki Disease appeared on the New York scene. We studied the epidemiology and risk factors ... and after Jane Newburger reported the success of intravenous gammaglobulin over 4 days of therapy, we reasoned that the same total dose (1gm/Kg) in a single large dose might be equally effective. It was ...

To summarise the high points in the trends I've seen over these 50 years, these are the ones I consider most significant: (1) the necessity of pediatric and surgical collaboration for precise diagnosis and appropriate medical and/or surgical management, (2) the clarification of diagnoses as improved techniques and the attendant improvement in operations as results of longterm follow ups emerged. (3) the importance of severe malformations in infancy and the increasing safety and efficacy of early repair, (4) the benefits of organizational cardiology and the committees whose work advanced the field, (5) the development of echocardiography in diagnosis and followup (6) the progress in invasive/therapeutic cardiology, (7) the appearance of Kawasaki Disease just as rheumatic fever continued on the decline, and the development of effective therapy, and (8) the continuing challenge of providing informed care longterm for adults with congenital heart disease."

—Engle MA 1994, quoted with permission.

Similar organisational change and growth occurred internationally, though most European centers [300] consisted of somewhat smaller groupings than the major divisions in North America. The Association of European Pediatric Cardiology was formed in the early 1960's, and generously included a few members from the United States and Canada. At annual spring meetings in enjoyable locations, ranging from Prague to Paris to Rhodes, there was a good exchange of knowledge, stimulated by polylingualism and hospitality. At a particularly happy meeting in Rhodes the late Bernhardt Landtmann of Helsinki spoke movingly of the growth of medical history, spreading from the nearby island of Cos to the present cardiac gathering in fellowship of the old world with the new.

By the time of the meeting of the Third World Congress of Pediatric Cardiology in Bangkok Thailand in 1989 it was clear that cardiologists around the world were approaching their common problems with similar tools and concepts, though with wide variations in staffing and facilities for research.

Geographic Cardiology

It would be invidious to try to name all the centers which have helped the discipline of pediatric cardiology grow and thrive, even if one had adequate scholarship to do so. Some advances, for example Doppler echocardiography, the major advance of the last 2 decades, has flourished in many widespread sites; and names from Lindsay Allan through David Sahn could be cited, covering much of the alphabet.

Other advances are clearly associated with one city, as is Marseilles with tetralogy of Fallot, or Tokyo with Kawasaki disease. Some might cavil at the inclusion of Capetown, where Barlow first clarified the syndrome of mitral valve prolopse, though probably most would agree with its inclusion for cardiac transplantation, pioneered by Christian Barnard. Despite the possibility of disagreement, we have chosen to mark some centers on the map in Figure 16, and assure the interested reader that at least one major contribution from each is in the text. Pediatric cardiology is a small but vibrant part of the global village of the modern world.

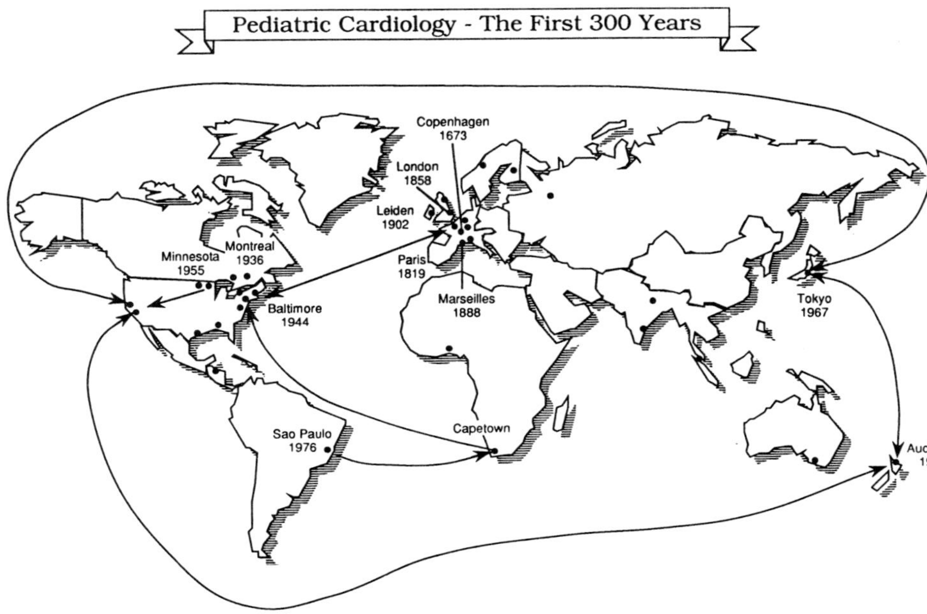

Fig 16—World Map showing some centers which have been part of the history of pediatric cardiology

The Child's World

In 1944, the year of the first Blalock Taussig shunt, Anne Frank was writing the last words in her diary. Eighty years earlier, in 1884, Mark Twain published the Adventures of Huckleberry Finn, while Fallot must have been preparing his extraordinary communication for the Marseilles medical journal. In 1750, while William Hunter was studying heart defects, there was rioting in Paris because the populace believed poor children were being kidnapped by members of the police [301].

In 1673, when Steno wrote of the malformed heart of a still born infant, little had been written for children, or about their lives. As books for children have grown, outdistancing even the burgeoning literature of pediatric cardiology, the child's own feelings about his heart remain as mysterious as in the time of della Robbia. One must hope that a history of pediatric cardiology written in the next century will contain more of the words and experiences of the children who have needed cardiac care, and in doing so, have touched all our lives and hearts.

ADDITIONAL REFERENCES AND NOTES

282. The ventricular septum of the heart. Wenink ACG, Oppenheimer-Dekker A, Moulaert AJ The Hague Martinius Nijhoff for Leiden U Press 1981.

283. Griswold HE, Bing RJ, Handelsman JC, Campbell J, Le Brun E. Physiologic studies in congenital heart disease. VII. Pulmonary arterial hypertension in congenital heart disease. Johns Hokins Hosp Bull 1949;84:76-78.

284. French H. A series of small points. Three clinical lectures. Lecture II Guys Hosp Gazette 1918;32:87 (reproduced in Circulation 1968;37:69 "50 years ago").

285. Moe DG, Guntheroth WG. Spontaneous closure of uncomplicated ventricular septal defect. Am J Cardiol 1987;60:674-678.

286. Martin GR, Perry LW, Ferencz C. Increased prevalence of ventricular septal defect: epidemic or improved diagnosis? Pediatrics 1989;83:200-203.

287. Kidd L, Driscoll DJ, Gersony WM et al. Second natural history study of congenital heart disease: Results of treatment of patients with ventricular septal defects. Circulation 1993; 87:138-151.

288. Neill CA, Clark EB. Tetralogy of Fallot: the first 300 years. Texas Heart Inst J 1994: in Press. December 1994.

289. Voisin M, Doan B, Elboury S et al. Extracardiac malformations in tetralogy of Fallot. Arch mal coeur vaiss 1989;82:689-692.

290. Taussig HB, Kallman CH, Nagel D et al. Long-time observations on the Blalock -Taussig operation VIII. 20-28 year follow-up on patients with tetralogy of Fallot. Johns Hopkins Med J 1975;137:13-19.

291. Kirklin JW, Karp RB. The tetralogy of Fallot from a surgical viewpoint. Philadelphia: WB Saunders 1970.

292. Gott VL. And it happened during our lifetime. Ann Thorac Surg 1993;55:1057-1064.

293. Shprintzen RJ, Goldberg RB, Young D, Wolford L. The velo-cardio-facial syndrome: a clinical and genetic analysis. Pediatrics 1981;67:167-172.

294. Freedom RM, Rosen FS, Nadas AS. Congenital cardiovascular disease and anomalies of the third and fourth pharyngeal pouch. Circulation 1972;46:165-172.

295. Holmes AF. An unusual anomaly of the heart Tr Edin Med Chi Soc 1824.

296. Abbott ME. Reexamination of the Holmes heart. Montreal Med J. July 1901.

297. Van Praagh R, Ongley PA, Swan HJC. Anatomic types of single or common ventricle in man:morphologic and geometric aspects of sixty necropsied cases. Am J Cardiol 1964;13:367-386.

298. Shineburne EA, Macartney FJ, Anderson RH. Sequential chamber localisation. Logical approach to diagnosis in congenital heart disease Br Heart J 1976;38:327-340.

299. Williams RG, Kennedy TL, Moller JH. Pediatric cardiology in the 1990's. J Am Coll Cardiol 1984;23:977-980.

300. Daniels O, Choussat A. La cardiologie pediatrique en Europe (editorial). Arch Mal Coeur Vaiss 1993;86:539-540.

301. Farge A, Revel J. The vanishing children of Paris. English Polity Press 1991.

CHAPTER 8

Developmental Era The 1990s and beyond

- Studies in Cardiac Development
- Preventive Approaches: Closing the Circle

"The fundamental question in relation to pathological embryos is that of heredity versus environment; and the subject of the causation of monsters is one of the dark pages in human history, associated as it is with our worst superstitions."

Florence R. Sabin in Franklin Paine Mall: the Story of a Mind. Johns Hopkins Press, 1934:305.[302]

"The great day will come when we learn how to prevent these birth defects rather than only to treat them."

Dr. Helen Taussig, 1973.

Introduction

Observations of the developing cardiovascular system date from antiquity. Aristotle pictured the beating heart in a chicken egg [303]. Leonardo DaVinci's drawings of the developing embryo foreshadowed the accurate description of the shape changes that accompany the development of an embryo to fetus to living animal [304].

In the modern era, the first detailed studies of the heart were made by German histologists and anatomists in the 19th century. The advances of the German school of His and Ludwig were made by scientists who employed the new techniques of microscopy and camera lucida drawings combined with wax plate reconstructions. The field of human embryology has its origins in the work of His [305].

By the turn of the century, it became clear that scientific advances required the expertise of more than one man and his students. Thus, arose the concept of a research institute that included facilities for collecting and preserving material and the intellectual environment for synthesis of data in an open and collaborative manner. These research institutes, "Hilfsinstitue" brought together expertise of scientists focused on a single organ or system. Many thrive even today:

The Neurological Institute of Vienna - Prof. Obersteiner
The Neural Histological Institute of Madrid - Prof. Ramon y Cajal
The Sackenberg Neurological Institute of Frankfort - Prof. Edinger
The Wistar Institute of Anatomy and Biology of Philadelphia - Prof. Greenman

This concept was extended to human embryology by Dr. Franklin Paine Mall, Professor of Anatomy at The Johns Hopkins School of Medicine [306]. Mall was a respected embryologist with an extensive collection of vertebrate embryos and some of the best examples of human embryos existing at the time. With F. Kiebel, another student of his, he wrote the first text of human embryology, Manual of Human Embryology, initially in German and later translated into English. Mall commented that "Human embryology is ... the most promising field in research in anatomy because we have in hand the best collection of human embryos." Then as now, the limiting factor for innovative projects was financial resources. Mall turned to one of the early benefactors of medical education and research, the Carnegie Foundation of Washington.

From its opening in 1913, the Research Institute for Embryology, supported by the Carnegie Institution of Washington D.C., was a keystone of human developmental research. Conceived, organized and begun by Mall, the Carnegie Institution became the center where the most thorough and detailed analysis of the human cardiovascular system was carried out. Many seminal advances in the study of human embryology in general and cardiovascular development in particular were made by members of the Carnegie faculty.

Dr. George L. Streeter was recruited from the University of Michigan where he was the professor of anatomy. He worked for the remainder of his career in the analysis of pathological as well as normal human embryos and succeeded Mall as the director of the institute. The Streeter Horizon stage series was the pioneering systematic analysis of human development, serving as the ground work for our current knowledge [307].

Experimental embryology also had strong beginnings at the Carnegie. Mall's concept was to combine the fields of pathology, clinical history, anthropology and teratology in his analysis of abnormal human embryos. For more than 50 years a string of research relevant to the cardiovascular system came from F. P. Mall, G. L. Streeter, M. Rawles, R. L. DeHaan, G. C. Rosenquist, F. J. Manasek, and H. Stalsberg.

Their individual contributions were often examples of the application of new techniques to old questions. Mary Rawles developed marking techniques with vital dyes to define the cell fate maps of the early blastoderm. Rosenquist and Stalsberg working with DeHaan used tritiated thymidine to define the cell origin of the cardiac mesoderm. Manasek used the new technique of transmission electron microscopy to describe the cellular components of the early embryonic heart.

Other laboratories contributed substantially to the developing heart. At the University of Michigan, Patten and Berry wrestled with the biomechanical forces that transformed the cardiac tube to a four chambered heart. In Europe, Z. Rychter at the Charles University in Prague, F. Orts-Llorca in Madrid, J. A. Los in Amsterdam and A. Oppenheimer-Dekker in Leiden, and M. V. delaCruz in Mexico City continued the process of description, analysis and elucidation of morphogenetic movements and mechanisms of cardiac organogenesis.

The record of progress in cardiac development is gauged by the symposia addressing the issues of the developing cardiovascular system. The first modern meeting focusing entirely on the developing heart occurred in Dayton Ohio in 1968, where Dr Oscar Jaffee convened the 41 investigators who were active in research of heart development [308]. Subsequent contributions came in 1978 at the March of Dimes meeting in the Grand Canyon organized by Glenn Rosenquist [309]. In 1979, a European meeting in Lausanne Switzerland was organized by Tomas Pexieder [310]. The continued progress is documented in a series of international seminars organized by A. Takao and held every 5 years in Tokyo [311-314]. Analysis of these accounts confirms that the paradigm used in the etiologic study of other diseases is applicable to the broad range of cardiovascular disease which has its origins in abnormalities of cardiovascular development.

Convergence of Disciplines

A synthesis of scientific disciplines contributed immeasurably to our understanding of the spectrum of human cardiac malformation and the evolution of medical and surgical care of children born with a heart defect. Now more than 100 years since the first major contributions to the descriptive embryology of the heart, it is clear that these disciplines combined with new scientific tools define the developmental era.

Pathology contributed the fundamental definition to the anatomy of heart defects. The seminal work of Dr Maude Abbott at McGill University in Montreal was the first systematic analysis of the clinical features of cardiac abnormalities and the pathologic anatomy [2]. Essential for the surgeon, pathologic description defined differences and similarities that provided important clues to the grouping of congenital cardiovascular malformations. Yet few areas have been more controversial than the discussions of nomenclature, particularly surrounding pathologic terminology and definitions [305,315]. But these discussions were valuable, helping us focus on the issues of anatomy. Now, from the perspective of years, we can look back on these sometimes fervent discussions and recognize their benefit. We can also anticipate similar discussion in the future about other topics, because it is the nature of discovery and reanalysis.

The epidemiologist defined the substrate of disease prevalence, the analysis of person, place and time [217]. From careful data analysis comes risk factors, not in themselves a cause of disease but rather valuable clues for analysis and validation in the laboratory and study design. Birth defect studies are distinct from traditional epidemiology [316].

The basic scientist's tools have expanded exponentially in the last two decades [314]. The boundaries of the cell and its matrix have yielded to the light and electron microscope, individual cell constituents to antibodies, and the human genome to dissection by molecular techniques. The environment of the developing heart, its functional capacity, biomechanical properties and systems control are integral to the assembly of the sophisticated self-sustaining pump.

Pediatric cardiologists have had a yin and yang relationship to the spectrum of a child's affliction. By the nature of their craft, they focused on the heart defect, aggressively developing new diagnostic techniques and surgical therapy but often neglecting the involvement of other systems. Perhaps to guard against the extraordinary risks taken in attempt to treat the previously untreatable, cardiologists and surgeons painted an idealistic picture for the child who survived the intricate heart surgery [317]. They left to others the chronic management of renal neurologic and skeletal anomalies.

Clinical pediatric cardiology contributed the careful analysis of cases, groups, associations and syndromes that are invaluable to the formal study of disease. These clinical clues are remarkable short cuts, much as the fortuitous linkage is to the molecular geneticist. There are numerous examples, but several are most pertinent because of the link to the molecular etiology.

The study of the conotruncal anomaly face syndrome by Takao and colleagues expanded the cluster of multi organ system defects [318]. The association of DiGeorge Syndrome with retinoic acid therapy defined a teratogen and clue to pathogenesis [319]. The story relating 22qll.2 deletion syndromes with multi-organ system defects vividly illustrates the importance of collaboration and integration by specialists of different disciplines [320].

As the *genetic dissection of defects* and dysmorphic syndrome progresses, precise description of mild phenotypic features becomes more important. Minor features like bifid uvula or deformed ear lobe with or without heart malformation may indicate a carrier state and the mildest phenotypic expression. The clinician needs improved techniques to define the 3-dimensional anatomical detail of the heart including the precise dimensions of the subpulmonic conal muscle, absence of the conal papillary muscle and the area of the membranous ventricular septum. Such studies will clarify the range of phenotypic expression and define the prevalence rate of defects so that we can understand the nature of penetrance of these defects.

From *descriptive embryology* comes the precise analysis of the primary shape changes of the embryonic heart [321]. The transition of the heart from a single muscle wrapped tube to a complex four chambered organ is the fundamental process of heart development. Descriptive embryology is the oldest of the developmental disciplines originating with the light microscope and camera lucida drawing, but new tools of the scanning electron microscope, quantitative morphology and immuno-histochemistry continue to provide structural definition to integrate information from molecular and cell biology.

Advances in the Mechanisms of Cardiovascular Development

The field of cardiac development has moved to a phase of intensive investigation of molecular mechanisms that regulate normal development. Progress is made with new tools. New tools of the developmental biologist, tools which were honed in studies of invertebrates, are applicable to the vertebrate heart. Recent developments added to this armamentarium include: retrovirus transfection, transgene and teratogen models.

The experimental data comes from in vivo models of heart development, primarily the chick embryo, that shares the morphologic characteristics of the human embryo during early development; in vitro organ and cell culture of mammalian embryos; and innovative computer models of cardiac cellular events. Animal models are integral to our understanding of cardiovascular development including: Drosophila for an understanding of patterning, zebra fish, transgenic mouse and spontaneous mutations.

Cardiac development is controlled by genetic and epigenetic (environmental) factors. The heart is not built from a blueprint, but rather takes shape guided by highly conserved phylogenetic mechanisms. Development is directed by morphoregulatory genes, regulated by feedback mechanisms that control growth, and integrated through biomechanical assembly of gene products. These events trigger the cascade of cell and tissue interactions that results in the four chambered heart.

There are 4 major developmental steps in the process of cardiovascular development. While clearly a continuous process, these steps include:

- Formation of the cardiac tube from the lateral cardiac mesoderm, situs and looping with segmental expression
- Elaboration of the myocardium
- Septation of the conotruncus, ventricles, atrioventricular canal and atria
- Genesis of the coronary and pulmonary vessels and connections

The multifaceted process of cardiac development remains a major challenge to embryologists and developmental biologists. At its simplest level, heart development is a biomechanical process that obeys the laws of physics. The heart is an example of precise spatial organization of tissue brought about by biomechanical forces. Energy is required for all steps in morphogenesis from uncoiling and transcription of DNA to each beat of the embryonic heart. While studies of gene expression are important in defining the genetic component of morphogenesis, the intervening steps of gene product assembly that produce a sarcomere, a myocyte, the myocardium, the cardiac loop and finally the four chambered heart are the crux of normal development. While the embryo is growing exponentially, the heart pumps blood to supply the embryo with nutrients and oxygen and to remove metabolic wastes.

Increasingly, specific molecular defects are being associated with pathogenetic cardiac disorders, giving rise to a new field of molecular epidemiology. With rapid advancement of genetics, molecular and cytogenetics, categorization of heart defects by single gene, polygene, chromosomal aberration and cytoplasmic inheritance would be revisited and challenged. Elucidation of mechanisms underlying abnormal meiosis, deletion or translocation will lead to final reduction in defects due to chromosomal anomaly.

Progress in Cardiovascular Development has not only provided information about congenital heart defects, but also expanded our understanding of the continuum of cardiovascular disease. Although abnormalities of cardiac development are most apparent as congenital defects, heart development is not just a child related issue.

More than 350 years ago, Sir Thomas Browne understood the importance of developmental events. In his treatise Religio Medici published in 1642, he wrote:

> *"And surely we are all of the computation of our age, and every man is some months elder than he bethinks him; for we live, move, have a being, and are subject to the actions of the elements, and the malice of diseases, in that other World, the truest Microcosm, the Womb of our Mother."*

Spectrum of Congenital Cardiovascular Malformations

Abnormal cardiovascular development is responsible for a broad spectrum of heart diseases with wide variability in clinical effects [322]. Most congenital cardiovascular malformations have their origins during primary morphogenesis and some forms of adult onset cardiovascular disease also arise during embryonic development.

As with most diseases, the severe end of the spectrum is easiest to recognize. Each of the most common severe defects has clear symptoms and natural or unnatural history. Subtle structural defects are less often recognized, and have fewer consequences on an individual's life. Bicuspid aortic valve is only symptomatic when infected or stenotic. Silent deviations in development may lead to abnormal mitral aortic continuity that has no influence on a person's health.

Congenital cardiovascular defect may be expressed in abnormal function. Ventricular muscle failure decades after successful tetralogy repair likely reflect an abnormality of the myocardium rather than the consequence of surgery. Likewise, arrhythmias are due to the underlying substrate of the conduction system and the complex process of excitation contraction coupling. Some forms of high blood pressure, coronary spasm have as a basis abnormalities in the functional integration of vascular resistance and blood flow control.

The patient's age when these defects are manifest also varies widely. As pediatric cardiologists, we focus on the defects of infancy, those anomalies that risk shortened live expectancy and death. Many abnormalities of cardiovascular development may only become apparent during adult life. Cardiogenesis and vasculogenesis are coordinated and interactive processes. Some types of hypertrophic and dilated cardiomyopathy may be traced to abnormalities in the way the myocardium is formed during the transition from a trabecular sponge-like chamber to compact dense ventricular walls. Hypertension may arise during embryonic development when the heart, devoid of autonomic innervation, perfuses the primitive cardiovascular system.

Abnormalities in the regulation of blood pressure in the pre-innervated circulation may persist into adult life. A congenitally bicuspid aortic valve often calcifies during adult life resulting in symptomatic aortic valve stenosis. A component of coronary artery disease may relate to abnormalities of vascular morphogenesis or control established during embryonic development.

THE SEARCH FOR ETIOLOGY AND PATHOGENESIS

With an increasing understanding of the process of normal cardiovascular development, the investigator turns to a delineation of the process of disease. Integral to this approach is an analysis of possible causes culled from analysis of human factors. Serendipity often plays a role in uncovering etiologic factors. But the systematic paradigm depends upon detailed analysis of human disease and the identification of risk factors [316].

Risk factors are statistical associations of environmental and or genetic components that occur non randomly in cases compared to controls. Risk factors do not determine cause. Rather they serve as clues for further biologic investigation and or as issues for population education. In no case should anyone accept this statistical association as evidence for cause, etiology or pathogenesis.

The single largest risk factor is a preoccurence of a congenital cardiovascular defect in the family. From this analysis comes some of the most intriguing information about congenital cardiovascular malformations that challenges the established ideas [320]. In the traditional view, the etiology of congenital cardiovascular malformations is multifactorial, a complex interaction of genetic and environmental causes. Continued analysis of an animal model, the Keeshond dog, originally thought to exhibit multifactorial inheritance of a conotruncal defect, clearly defined that the mechanism is a single major gene defect [323]. In humans, measures of pre-occurrence risk challenge this explanation for some of the most common defects.

Identifying the etiology and pathogenesis has been difficult because of the large number of anatomically distinct congenital cardiovascular defects with varying clinical consequences. A thorough understanding of the anatomic characteristics of congenital cardiovascular defects is essential to medical and surgical management. However, classification of heart defects by anatomic features may obscure developmental relationships. For the purposes of etiologic analysis, clustering defects by potential pathogenetic mechanisms has been fruitful. This organization of defects forms a conceptual background for analysis, and provides diagnostic groups of adequate size for comparison [212,214].

Syndromic Associations. In addition to the link between DiGeorge Syndrome and CATCH22, there is a crescendo of insight into the genomic abnormalities associated with cardiovascular syndromes. In Marfan syndrome the underlying molecular defect in fibrillin can be correlated with the pathogenesis of the cardiovascular changes in the aortic wall and mitral valve. Holt-Oram now is identified to a gene locus on chromosome 12. Alagille syndrome gene maps to chromosome 20. This association is particulary important because the Alagille gene is that same gene that codes for the protein ES130. ES130 is a determinant of cell lineage during early differentiation of the heart tube and instruction to cells that will become the myocardium.

Frontiers of Diagnosis and Therapy

Understanding of some congenital cardiovascular malformations and late onset heart disease is sufficiently advanced for planning of diagnosis and therapy.

FETAL DIAGNOSIS

Ultrasound has provided a dramatic new window on the developing human. There are more than 4 million pregnancies in the United States each year. At least 25% or 1,000,000 women have a fetal ultrasound study and in 50,000 there is a detailed fetal echocardiogram. The fetal cardiovascular studies are done as early as 10 weeks post conception. The early diagnosis of chromosomal and metabolic abnormalities can be accomplished by amniocentesis. From these studies, clinical decisions are made about intervention and the future of the pregnancy [324].

There is a need for additional basic information on the human fetus at these early stages. In spite of decades of research, comparatively little is known about the gross anatomy of the fetal heart and circulation and the physiology, biochemistry, metabolism, cellular morphology and pharmacology of the human cardiovascular system. Indeed, even the most basic descriptive information on the human embryo and fetal cardiovascular system is lacking.

Fetal therapy for cardiovascular disorder is underway despite the relative lack of basic information. Preclampsia is pathogenetically related to the failure of placental spiral arteries to transform from thick walled high resistance vessels to thin walled low resistance conduits. In a recent controlled clinical trial, maternal fetal pairs were treated with aspirin as a method of facilitating the muscular arterial wall changes. The future holds promise for other treatment mechanisms using small peptides that cross the placenta and can be targeted to fetal tissue.

MYOCARDIAL DISEASE

Rapid progress is being made in defining the genomic abnormalities in some forms of myocardial disease. Hypertrophic cardiomyopathy and X-linked dilated cardiomyopathy have defined abnormal gene loci. Increasingly, as molecular biology advances, cardiovascular disease has become a continuum. The paradigm is the study of cardiomyopathy.

Two generations of intensive investigation of the natural history, physiology, morphology, and family incidence of hypertrophic cardiomyopathy have culminated in the definition of specific genetic defects. Thus, a cardiac disorder which usually becomes manifest in late childhood or early adult life is due to a problem predating conception. The next challenges focus on the pathogenesis of these defects.

We must understand the temporal spatial expression of the gene groups and the mechanisms from myocyte determination to the fabric of the myocardium. This can only be done by studying expression libraries raised from human embryo and fetal myocardium obtained at precise points in development. These have broad application to the treatment of human disease. The prospects of clinical regulating myocyte proliferation are very real. The promise is for therapy that will activate the quiescent non-replicating ventricular myocyte to re-populate the fibrosed and damaged heart. This important goal, too, depends upon defining the cell regulatory mechanisms in human embryo and fetal myocardium.

HYPERTENSION, STROKE AND CORONARY ARTERY DISEASE

The heart and circulation begin to function long before there is any renal or brain control of hemodynamics. The pathogenesis of some forms of hypertension likely occurs in the integration of layered tissue and central nervous system control mechanisms during fetal development. Studies of gene expression and vascular regulatory control will define the sequential development of cardiovascular homeostasis and interrelationship to environment. There is great potential for therapeutic intervention in a disordered developmental process.

In spite of billions of dollars spent each year on the treatment of coronary artery disease, we have only basic descriptive information on the embryology of the myocardial circulation. The mechanisms of coronary vasculogenesis are unknown. Likewise, the regulatory mechanisms of vascular endothelial biology are unexplored. Progress in defining the fundamental liability for coronary vascular disease requires a understanding of the development of the human coronary vascular bed and its physiology, biochemistry and regulatory control.

CLOSING THE CIRCLE THAT LEADS TO PREVENTION

In her later years, Dr. Helen B. Taussig, the founder of modern pediatric cardiology, sought the root cause of the cardiac defects that she had devoted her life to treating. Her hypothesis was that many if not most congenital cardiac defects reflected expression of genetic causes [325]. At the time, her ideas were greeted with skepticism since few thought that a single gene could be responsible for a complex defect like Tetralogy of Fallot. However, as we advance our knowledge of cardiovascular development, we will uncover the etiology and pathogenesis of a broad range of disease and the therapy that can lead to prevention.

ADDITIONAL REFERENCES

302. Sabin FR. Franklin Paine Mall, the Story of a Mind. Baltimore: Johns Hopkins Press, 1934.
303. Adelmann, HB. Marcello Malpighi and the evolution of embryology. Ithaca NY: Cornell Univ Press 1966; vol 2:729-781, vol 3: 1300-1511.
304. O'Malley CD, Saunders JBdeCM. Leonardo da Vinci on the human body. New York: Henry Schuman, 1952.
305. O'Rahilly R. One hundred years of human embryology. Issues Rev. Teratol. 1988;4:81-128.
306. Mall FP. A plea for an institute of human embryology. JAMA 1913;60:1599-1601.
307. O'Rahilly R, Muller F. Developmental stages in human embryos. Baltimore: Carnegie Institution of Washington, Publication 637, 1987.
308. Jaffee, OC. Cardiac development with special reference to congenital heart disease. Dayton, Ohio: University of Dayton Press, 1970.
309. Rosenquist GC, Bergsma D. Morphogenesis and malformation of the cardiovascular system. New York, Alan R. Liss, National Foundation-March of Dimes. Birth Defects: Original Article Series, Vol XIV, No.7,1978.
310. Pexieder T. Mechanisms of cardiac morphogenesis and teratogenesis. New York, Raven Press, 1981.
311. VanPraagh R, Takao A. Etiology and morphogenesis of congenital heart disease. Mount Kisco, NY: Futura, 1980.
312. Nora JJ, Takao A. Congenital heart disease: Causes and progress. Mount Kisco, NY: Futura Publishing, 1985.
313. Clark EB, Takao A. Developmental cardiology: Morphogenesis and function. Mount Kisco, NY: Futura Publishing, 1990.
314. Clark EB, Markwald RR, Takao A. Developmental mechanisms of heart disease. Mount Kisco, NY: Futura Publishing, 1994.
315. Anderson RH. Terminology. In: Anderson RH, Macartney FJ, Shinebourne EA, Tynan M, eds. Paediatric Cardiology. Edinburgh: Churchill Livingstone 1987:65-82.
316. Clark EB. Epidemiology of congenital cardiovascular malformations. In: Emmanouilides GC, Riemenschneider TA, Allen H,Gutgesell HP eds. Heart Disease in Infants, Children and Adolescents, 5th Edition. Baltimore: Williams and Wilkins, 1994.
317. Moller JH. Fifty years of pediatric cardiology and challenges for the future. Circulation 1994; 89:2479-2483.
318. Takao A, Momma K, Kondoh C, Ando M, Shimizu T, Burn J, Matsuoka R. Conotruncal anomaly face syndrome. In: Clark EB, Markwald RR, Takao A eds. Developmental mechanisms of heart disease. Mt. Kisco NY: Futura Publishing 1994.
319. Lammer EJ, Opitz JM. The DiGeorge anomaly as a developmental field defect. Am J Med Genet 1986;2 (suppl):113-127.
320. Burn J. Human models of cardiac defects. In: Clark EB, Markwald RR, Takao A eds. Developmental mechanisms of heart disease. Mt. Kisco NY: Futura Publishing 1994.
321. Ferrans VJ, Rosenquist G, Weinstein C. Cardiac morphogenesis. New York: Elsevier, 1985.

322. Moller JH, Allen HD, Clark EB, Dajani AS, Golden A, Hayman LL, Lauer RM, Marmer EL, McAnulty JH, Oparil S, Strauss AW, Taubert KA, Wagner A. Report of the Task Force on Children and Youth. Circulation 1993;88:2479-2486.

323. Patterson DF, Pexieder T, Schnarr WR, Navratil T, Alaili R. A single major gene defect underlying cardiac conotruncal malformations interferes with myocardial growth during embryonic development: studies in the CTD line of keeshond dogs. Am J Hum Genet 1993;52:388-397.

324. Hansen JT, Sadek JR. Fetal research. Science 1989;246:775-779.

325. Taussig HB. Evolutionary origin of cardiac malformations. JACC 1988;12:1079-1086.

CHAPTER 9

Ethics and Public Policy The frontiers of cardiovascular treatment and prevention

- Therapy: changing ethical issues
- Molecular biology, screening, the fetal heart

The heart has a central, nearly mythical, place in our modern society. Human history is replete with references dating from antiquity. The Egyptians placed special emphasis on the heart. At death, they separated the heart from the body and enshrined it in a vessel of clay. The Aztec's human sacrifices involved removing a beating heart thus, celebrating its seeming essence of life. The heart is no less central in Judaeo-Christian culture, producing ethical and public policy dilemmas.

In the Middle Ages, the heart and human body were the center of ecclesiastical turmoil. During the centuries dominated by the Catholic Church, dissection of the human body was banned by Papal decree. Longstanding fear and awe proscribed operating on the human heart and influenced generations of surgeons. Altman emphasized the reluctance of surgeons to attempt cardiac repairs in a quote from Dr. Stephen Paget in 1897, "Surgery of the heart has probably reached the limits set by Nature to all surgery: no new method, and no new discovery can overcome the natural difficulties that attend a wound of the heart." [326]. The first attempts at cardiac surgery were driven by the urgency of injury from trauma of war and personal confrontations. Even as late as the 1930s there was strong professional interdiction against operating on the heart. Yet, in spite of the prevailing ethical constraints, talented physicians and surgeons pursued the dream of repairing the beating heart.

Beginning with the closed procedures and extending through deep hypothermia, crossed circulation and the early heart lung machine, pioneers including Blalock, Glenn, Gross, Gibbon, Waterston, Debakey, Lillehei and Mustard, produced a series of spectacular advances preserving life and prolonging survival of infants and children born with congenital cardiovascular anomalies [4, 12, 13]. Certainly, these teams of surgeons and cardiologists struggled with the incalculable risks weighed against the natural history of certain death.

Therapy: Changing Ethical Questions

In the last 50 years there has been a crescendo of ethical conflicts changing as society came to grips with technology and the scientific process that spawns advances in medical and surgical care. One area of contention was the use of animals in medical research and training. Arising in the late 19th century in England, the anti-vivisectionist movement strove to abolish animal research [327]. A particularly poignant confrontation occurred in Baltimore in the early 1950's when legislation to ban animal use was brought to the City Council. The opponents to animal research were quashed when Dr. Taussig paraded before the Council members a group of children who were alive because they had a Blalock Taussig shunt. Anna, once described by Alex Haller as "just a dog with no pedigree" [328], also played a role. She became celebrated in the press and in a portrait, as the first successful survivor of that operation.

The use of animals in cardiovascular research remains a point of contention between investigators and those who deem all experimentation morally and ethically unacceptable.

WHO SHOULD BE OPERATED ON?

Care for the child with a congenital cardiovascular malformation was largely determined by family socioeconomic status and residence. Initially, those children who arrived in Baltimore in the early days of the Blalock Taussig era were middle class or higher, with highly motivated parents intent on doing everything feasible for their child. The training of cardiac teams and development of additional cardiac centers distributed across the U.S now allows for access to care even for children in remote farming communities and large diverse urban areas.

Initially, children with chromosomal anomalies like Down syndrome were deemed inappropriate for surgery. But, as the outcome became clear, most centers in the United States aggressively treat these children. The same is not true in other countries. In some centers in Europe, there is a strong inclination against surgical intervention.

As medical resources are rationed in response to economic pressures, outcome analysis will play an increasing role in management decisions. Three long term issues must be considered: benefit to the child, the parents and society.

Who will be treated and how long? Central to these issues is an appraisal of benefit offered and risk encountered by children who have surgical repair. In simple terms, the infant should receive treatment to ensure or restore an active happy life, with the minimum of pain and distress involved in the remedy. The pediatric cardiologist must imagine how he or she would wish to be treated if in the infant's place. This seemingly simple process is hampered by a fundamental lack of knowledge about the true prognosis of many complex defects, particularly those where the cardiac anomaly is part of a syndrome affecting many different organ systems. Lurking in each cardiologist's mind is the horror of an infant submitted to multiple cardiac operations, invasive procedures and prolonged intensive care and ventilator support for a defect that is uniformly fatal in the first year of life.

For some cardiac defects aggressive medical and surgical care has been profoundly beneficial. On this end of the spectrum are tetralogy of Fallot and transposition of the great vessels. Children with these defects have lived longer and more productive lives with the advent of surgical care. We recognize however, that they are not cured of their defect. Each may have has a lingering morbidity and mortality which is expressed later in life [317].

For defects at the other end of the spectrum, like hypoplastic left heart syndrome and complex single ventricle, the benefit is less clear. Over the last 15 years, hypoplastic left heart syndrome, a nearly uniformly fatal defect, has been the focus of a series of palliative surgical procedures aimed at rescuing infants. Surgical therapy was first attempted by Doty in the 1970s and developed by Norwood, whose name is now used as an eponym for a complex staged operation to separate the systemic and pulmonary blood flow.

There is considerable discussion and debate as to the ethical treatment for this common and lethal defect. Some suggest that vigilant fetal monitoring and early in utero diagnosis may lead to early recognition, the option for elective therapeutic abortion and a subsequent reduction in live born prevalence for this agonizing defect. Others feel strongly that their team's outcome with the Norwood procedure or infant cardiac transplantation is at least as good as the outcome for other complex defects. They reason that it is no longer proper to discuss with the parents of an otherwise normal neonate the option for compassionate care.

With this therapeutic uncertainty, the pediatric cardiologist must often counsel parents and face the arduous task of informing, educating, without being overly directive. Yet it is nearly impossible to articulate a complex situation without introducing one's own bias. These recommendations and parental decisions are not made in isolation. Family and friends are often aware of the nature of the disease and results in well publicized cases. The press has reported the drama surrounding these uncertain courses of therapy. Baby Jesse born with hypoplastic left heart syndrome received a new heart transplanted from an infant with anencephaly. Baby Amy's parents chose to spare her from the agony and heroic measures of repeated surgery. Each of these cases drew national and international coverage, and a range of public comment from support to rage [329].

The pendulum of medical therapy swings slowly through a broad arc that begins with glorious reports of outcome and follows with complications and eventually questioning of the place of the operation itself. Often the nature of the experiments were not obvious to parents or medical participants. The true value of surgical intervention is apparent only with time.

As we move to a health care system that is driven in large part by cost and outcome, how will we assess the benefit to society? Some children with complex syndromic heart disease have multi-system involvement often with severe mental retardation. Cardiac surgical procedures may palliate their condition, but are not an assurance of long survival or productive life. Will the infant with a small likelihood of surviving to become an adult who contributes to the economy of society be relegated to medical treatment rather than expensive surgical palliation? The Baby Doe controversy has led to a series of rulings maintaining that the preservation of life and well being of the child are a paramount societal good, outweighing any consideration of becoming a productive member of society.

The Molecular Genetics of Heart Disease: who has it and how much do they have?

These current quandaries about benefit to the individual and society are modest compared to the ethical dilemmas to be faced in the era of molecular diagnosis [330]. With continued progress in the human embryology, diagnosis of abnormal DNA, cell manipulation and gene therapy are on the therapeutic horizon. How do we balance the technology with the rights of the living children and adults and those yet to be born? Abnormal genes are a major component of congenital cardiovascular malformations. Rapid progress is being made in defining the human genome and the specific deletions and substitutions responsible for a wide range of cardiovascular disease and more are defined each month. At most recent count, the genomic basis of more than 70 defects with primary or secondary cardiac involvement is known.

CATCH22 Syndrome is a particularly illustrative example. The deletion of chromosome 22 q 11 locus is associated with field defect of branchial arch mesenchyme affecting the face, thymus, parathyroids and conotruncal region of the heart. At the center of this region, the TUPLE 1 gene deletions have been identified in pedigrees with reoccurrence of conotruncal defects.

In these complex cases, there are great problems that defy simplistic explanations. The appropriately called "myth of genetic determination" fails to identify the epigenic factors that participate in the complex biomechanical development of the heart. In the best case, the genotype produces the phenotype in a 1:1 relationship. In other conditions, this direct relationship does not hold true, because this simple formulation ignores the issues of phenotypic variability. Identifying the gene does not necessarily predict the phenotype. In one CATCH 22 family, the mother has a sub-mucous cleft palate, two daughters have sub-mucous cleft and tetralogy of Fallot, and a son is unaffected by all measures except that he shares their speech pattern. Mother and daughter's speech is produced in part by the sub-mucous cleft, the son because he has learned to talk like the rest of the family. When asked, he says he talks "the way everyone in my family talks."

A range of phenotypic variability is encountered in other pedigrees. For the past ten years, we have been studying the phenotypic variability in families of children with hypoplastic left heart syndrome. Approximately 50% have no identified abnormality, but in the others there is a range of defects from mild bicuspid aortic valve, through severe aortic valve stenosis and coarctation of the aorta. A powerful genetic defect can produce highly lethal disease with little phenotypic variation when fully expressed: yet in some pedigrees shared genetic abnormalities can produce a wide range of phenotypic defects. Similar variability is found among families with long QT syndrome associated with sudden death, and hypertrophic cardiomyopathy.

The search for at risk individuals: As the genetic basis of congenital heart disease is unraveled, there is a powerful drive to search for individuals at risk. Why? Because congenital cardiovascular malformations account for the largest portion of infant mortality from congenital defects. Cardiac defects are 5 times more prevalent than cystic fibrosis. It may prove that 50% of congenital cardiac defects are either autosomal dominant or recessive. Then 1 in 10 individuals possess one or other gene for a cardiac defect compared to 1/20 for cystic fibrosis.

The financial cost of congenital heart disease is substantial. Combined medical and surgical treatment for an individual child may cost more than $150,000; yet the value of successful treatment can be immeasurable in human terms, and as a paradigm of beneficence and societal good.

Who Should Be Tested? When? and Why? As we approach the time when routine testing is possible for the carrier state of heart disease in general and congenital cardiovascular malformation in particular, we must develop policies and procedures that will define and protect the rights of the individual in the face of society's pressures to reduce health care costs.

There is no current consensus on testing for the carrier state, with a few rare exceptions such as Tay Sachs or thalassemia, diseases which are either uniformly lethal or accompanied by prolonged morbidity and reduced life expectancy. The few agreed tenets include that testing should be:

- voluntary
- confidential
- restricted to specific indications
- directed to the best interests of family and society

It is generally agreed that voluntary testing implies that there is no social or financial pressure brought to bear on the family. The results should be confidential between the physician and patient or parent. Acceptable indications include major questions involving decisions on treatment or family planning. Testing should not be done simply to protect a physician or health care provider from "missing" a defect or disorder.

When should the testing be done? Preconception or during the pregnancy? The specialist pediatric cardiologist will have only a limited contact with the families and individuals who are gene carriers. Thus, except for reoccurrence risk counseling after a child is born with a defect, it is not the pediatric cardiologist who will be advising about this type of screening.

The largest pool at risk are those carriers who are only beginning their reproductive life. If economical and reliable tests were available, should every high school senior be screened for a battery of genetic risk including cardiac defects, coronary artery disease, cardiomyopathy and cancers? Alternatively, screening could be part of preconception counseling.

Post conception screen depends on accurate phenotypic identification in utero and raises the possibility of therapy or termination of the pregnancy. There is also the opportunity to make phenotypic diagnosis in utero and adequately determine the fetuses heart defect. This in its own right produces a series of ethical dilemmas including the acceptance of termination and the accuracy of diagnosis. Confirmation of a genetic defect would require either analysis of a chorionic villous sample that carries a risk of 1% for spontaneous abortion or later amniocentesis.

The advantage is defining the affected fetus with the opportunity for intervention. These could be innovative techniques ranging from somatic cell engineering by construct insertion injected into the fetus at a critical point in development to peptide induced regulation of gene products.

FETAL TISSUE AS TREATMENT FOR HUMAN DISEASE

The goal for the next generation of pediatric cardiologists must be expanded to the prevention of cardiovascular disease. This calls for new and increased information on the basic biology of heart development. The paradigm for the study of human disease is well established. While many questions can initially be approached in animal models including transgenic constructs and knockouts and computer simulations, the cardiovascular scientist must also study human development in the embryo and fetus.

The use of human fetal tissue in the treatment of disease is another area of controversy. Pioneering work in the treatment of neurologic disease like Parkinsonism by fetal tissue transplantation into the basal ganglia, and therapy for retinitis pigmentosa by transplant of human fetal retinal cells into the affected individuals eyes, are the brave new world of therapy. Similar process can be extended to the heart and circulation.

As a cardiologist it grieves me each time I send a child with a dilated cardiomyopathy for heart transplantation. I wonder would it not be far better to keep the valves, coronaries and autonomic nervous system intact and supplement the myocardium with a fresh group of myocytes. Fetal myocyte transfer is now possible in laboratory modes.

Human fetal tissue research in general and fetal transplantation research in particular have been a flash point in the United States. The ethical construct for tissue use is clear and well established pivoting on informed consent, lack of coercion and financial gain, and anonymity. Still, the issue is contentious and a focus of the Right to Life movement and religious conservatives. For nearly 12 years, US federal polity banned the NIH support of fetal tissue transplantation research. This prohibition was lifted in 1992, soon after the inauguration of President Clinton.

The battle is now being carried to the other public arenas. Voluntary health organizations, like the American Heart Association, are under pressure to restrict funding of research on tissue obtained from medical terminations of pregnancy. The power of these special interest groups will likely influence what should be decisions made on the basis of scientific value balanced with the preservation of the rights of the individuals involved.

Not unlike the struggle for legitimate use of animals in cardiovascular research, there is an additional challenge to assure the use of human fetal tissue in the definition of disease and eventual therapy. These indeed will be interesting times.

ADDITIONAL REFERENCES

326. Altman LK. Who Goes First? New York: Random House, 1987.

327. Loeb JM, Hendee WR, Smith SJ, Schwartz MR. Human vs animal rights. JAMA 1989;262:2716-2720.

328. Haller JA Jr. Anna, Vivien, and the King of Cyan (osis). John Hopkins Med J. 1975;137:55-56.

329. Vuillemot L: The fate of Baby Amy. New York Times Magazine, September 25, 1988: 39.

330. Andrews LB, Fullarton JE, Holtzman NA, Motulsky AG. Assessing genetic risks: Implications for health and social polity. Washington DC: National Academy Press, 1994.

INDEX

A

B

C

D

E

F

G

H

IJ

K

L

M

N

O

P

QR

S

T

UV

WXYZ